JANE PATTERSON, M.D., F.A.C.O.G. is a
graduate of Chatham College in Pittsburgh,
Pennsylvania, and of the University of Pittsburgh School of Medicine. She is board certified
in obstetrics and gynecology, and is presently in
private practice in Glendale, California. She is
co-author, with Lynda Madaras, of WOMAN-
CARE: A GYNECOLOGICAL GUIDE TO
YOUR BODY, available from Avon Books.

LYNDA MADARAS is a freelance writer and
editor, and co-authored WOMANCARE with
Jane Patterson. She is currently working on a
novel and lives in Los Angeles, California.

W9-CYG-859

Other Avon Books by
Jane Patterson, M.D. and Lynda Madaras

WOMANCARE: A GYNECOLOGICAL GUIDE TO YOUR BODY

WOMAN/ DOCTOR

THE EDUCATION OF JANE PATTERSON, M.D.

Jane Patterson and Lynda Madaras

AVON
PUBLISHERS OF BARD, CAMELOT, DISCUS AND FLARE BOOKS

WOMAN/DOCTOR: THE EDUCATION OF JANE PAT-
TERSON, M.D. is an original publication of Avon Books.
This work has never before appeared in book form.

The names of most of the people and places in this book
have been changed to protect the innocent and the guilty.
The details of the incidents described have been rearranged
and reshaped to protect the anonymity of the people involved. Despite this camouflaging, the book holds to the es-
sential truth.

AVON BOOKS
A division of
The Hearst Corporation
959 Eighth Avenue
New York, New York 10019

Copyright © 1983 by Lynda Madaras
Published by arrangement with the author
Library of Congress Catalog Card Number: 83-90628
ISBN: 0-380-83063-9

First Avon Printing, July, 1983

AVON TRADEMARK REG. U. S. PAT. OFF. AND IN
OTHER COUNTRIES, MARCA REGISTRADA, HECHO EN
U. S. A.

Printed in the U. S. A.

WFH 10 9 8 7 6 5 4 3 2 1

For the chief, who taught me how to care; for Betty, who taught me how to feel.

J.P.

For the friends who kept me going during the writing of this book (in alphabetical order, because there is no other way to weigh it): Al (Sr. and Jr.), Alma, Anita, Area, Beth, Betty, BHC, BV, Carol, Carole, Claire, Claudia, Elizabeth, Eric, George, Grace, Hannah, Harold, Jane, Jared, Jean, Jeannene, Jeff, Ken (both of you), Mag, Norma, the Pams, Patti, Richard, Sarah, Skeeter, Susan, Tony, Walter. Thanks to all of you.

L.M.

ONE

THE RAYS were coming in my window. The sun was shining its southern California best. The birds were singing in the palm trees just off the freeway. It was Los Angeles, January 1967, and it was coming up on the end of my second year of residency training.

I woke with the sun full on my face, savoring it; and the fact that I had anything left inside with which to savor sunshine has to be some sort of testament to the human spirit, because six and a half years at this business of becoming a doctor had pretty much dried the sap out of my veins.

Those first four years of medical school cannot have been as bad as I remember them, but I'll never know for sure because, to this day, I can barely pierce the droning grey monotony that hangs over my memory of those years long enough to find out. All that I have left of those years is a string of shapeless, indeterminate days and nights spent memorizing a million multisyllabic Latin names for every bit of muscle, bone and tissue in the human body. And I was swimming upstream against the current the whole time, a woman in medical school in the early sixties. But maybe I exaggerate and complain too much, making, as always, too much of things. After all, it wasn't a *million* names. Still, someone did once tell me that you add forty thousand new words to your vocabulary in medical school, or maybe it was

1

twenty thousand. Anyhow, it was a lot of words, but even the deadening boredom of all that rote memorization might have been bearable except that it took up so much time. Medical school, anatomy lab and hospital rotations became my entire reality, and the rest of life just sort of faded away as I was swallowed up by a world so insular that I was only vaguely aware of the extent of my isolation.

Sometimes now I'll be sitting around over a bottle of wine with friends, the ones who aren't doctors, and they'll be struck with sudden fits of nostalgia, recalling the early sixties: the Twist, the pop songs that passed right by me, Elvis Presley, Marilyn Monroe, space shots. Or, in a more serious vein, the civil rights movement—sit-ins; Selma, Alabama, and the Freedom Riders; Martin Luther King.

"Of course, Marilyn Monroe," I'll offer. "She died then, didn't she? Suicide or something, wasn't it?"

My friends groan. "Where were you?" Humming bits of early Beatles tunes that I never heard until they became Muzak in hospital elevators, they want to know what I was doing when JFK died. Studying, surely, but I don't really remember. I'm as entertaining as a clam at these nostalgia games. I can offer little more than my recollection of the time Bill Mazeroski hit a home run at the bottom of the ninth and the Pittsburgh Pirates had their first pennant since 1925. And I remember that only because Forbes Field, which was the Pirates' home field back then, was en route from the medical school to my house, and thanks to the big game I was stuck in a six-hour traffic jam the night before a pathology exam.

When I wasn't studying, I was at the hospital or in anatomy lab doing gruesome and disgusting things to grey, decaying cadavers, pickled livers and other dead things. My world narrowed; old friends sort of faded away. They were leading normal, regular lives, and when I did make time to visit them, it always seemed that the most interesting thing that had happened to me lately would be something on the order of a fascinating case of facial cancer that was eating away the upper lip and half of the nose of some poor old man I'd encountered in clinic—which is hardly the sort of thing you can trot out in casual conversation. Besides, I reeked of formaldehyde from being in anatomy lab all the time, and my friends were always sniffing about wanting to know what that peculiar odor was.

Very early on, my fantasies of being the great doctor, healing the sick and helping stamp out disease, which were what had gotten me into medicine in the first place, began to recede into a dim and unforeseeable future. But, somehow, I made it through. I even managed to graduate near the top of my class. Having proved I could ovulate and think at the same time, an idea without a large following in those days, I was eligible for a prestigious internship, so I went off to Prestigious U for my internship year—the year of the walking dead, which is even worse than medical school. Then after the internship, for those who are going to specialize, there are two to eight years of residency training depending on the speciality. Following a prolonged and schizophrenic bout of indecision, I chose a three-year residency in obstetrics and gynecology, known in the business as OB/GYN, or "obie, gine." But I had to leave Prestigious U to do it. The head of the residency program there was widely quoted as having said that he supposed one day he'd be forced to take a woman or a black into the program and, if so, he'd take the black. I decided I needed cleaner air to breathe, and I interviewed elsewhere.

It came down to two choices. One was another prestigious university hospital, a citadel of academic medicine, where I was interviewed by three suave, sartorial splendors with three-hundred-dollar suits and wavy silver pompadours, all Big Men in Medicine, who let me know that they might take me into their program even though I was a woman. The other was a not-so-prestigious, nonuniversity hospital where I was interviewed by three fat men with balding heads and without big reputations, who let me know they wanted me *because* I was a woman. I immediately fell in love with the three fat men and would have followed them to the bowels of hell if that was where their hospital had been; but luckily, it was right here in Los Angeles.

My residency was much better than what had come before, and by the middle of the second year, I was beginning to notice things like the sun shining on my face again, and to think I might actually survive my medical training. In six short months I'd begin my third and final year of residency training. After that, I'd be . . . well, I didn't really know what I'd be, but I'd be finished. I would be fully trained.

It would be years before I would know what it had cost me.

I was working in the operating room on that sunny day in January, which suited me just fine. Surgery was one of the things I truly loved about being a doctor: the order and ritual of it, the intensity of the concentration, the drama and delicacy of the work. I still love it, but then it was a newer love, and more than that, it appealed to me emotionally. It was so clean-cut, so straightforward. Someone came in sick, I'd open her up, cut out the sickness, and send her on her way. It was all so unambiguous, so black and white, so unlike the shades of grey that colored the rest of my life.

My last operation that day was with the chief of staff, as his first assistant. I'd operated with him before, and it was fascinating to watch him work. He had squat, square hands with thick, stubby fingers, more like a butcher's than the long and elegant con-

cert pianist's hands you'd imagine for a virtuoso surgeon. But when he worked, they moved deftly, with a
surprising delicacy. It was like watching a fat lady un-
expectedly light on her feet, dancing with incongru-
ous grace. In the middle of the operation, he turned
the case over to me, assuming the role of first assistant. "Good job, Doctor," he told me afterwards,
snapping off his gloves, and I went off to dinner walking tall. It wasn't every day that the chief of staff
turned a case over to a second-year resident.

I was on call in obstetrics that night, which meant
spending the night at the hospital on one of the buz-
zard-feather mattresses in the on-call room and being
wakened twenty times, but I was feeling too good to
mind. By midnight, things had slowed down. There
were only a few women in the labor suite. It didn't
look as though any of them would deliver for several
hours, which in the unpredictable matter of birth
means absolutely nothing. Still, I was entertaining
the notion that I might actually get some sleep when
the nasal twang of the page operator's voice came at
me through the loudspeaker in the corridor. I was
wanted in Admitting.

Normally, a page to Admitting isn't anything terribly urgent. It's not like being paged to the emergency
room or getting a STAT call. Usually it's just some
snarl in the hospital's red tape—someone has managed to admit the wrong patient to the wrong room
on the wrong day, and they want you to come down
and untangle the mess.

But obstetrics is a bit different. The first-year resident handles routine admissions in OB. He isn't supposed to call for the second-year resident unless
there's a real problem. Even so, I wasn't too concerned. Howie Greenspan, the new first-year
resident, was on duty in Admitting. Howie was a replacement for one of the first-year residents who'd
been dragged off by the army. You had to wonder

about anyone who was floating around free and un-employed in the middle of his first year of residency, and it wasn't too hard to see why someone might have let Howie go before the end of his first year. He'd arrived on the ward a couple of months ago like a haystack on fire. He had vast amounts of energy and an earnest, eager air. He also had a gift for creating chaos out of order and an intern's flair for wild-eyed diagnosis. If Howie heard hoofbeats thundering by his window, he'd have concluded that a zebra had just run by. He'd already panicked half a dozen patients with his dazzling leaps of logic, conjuring up all sorts of pregnancy complications rarely seen outside the confines of a medical textbook. They had him on a tight rein. He wasn't to so much as speak to a patient, let alone run any tests, without first discussing his diagnostic theories with someone senior to him.

So I wasn't exactly overcome with a sense of urgency about Howie's paging me. Still, the law of averages being what it was, Howie was bound to run into a bona fide medical emergency sooner or later, so I responded promptly to the page and hurried over to Admitting.

As I came around the corner, I heard the voice of a woman just this side of hysteria.

"It's coming. It's coming. The baby is coming!" she was yelling.

I met Howie in the corridor just outside her room.

"Prolapsed cord. Heartbeat's irregular and down below sixty. I've notified Delivery," he told me in a single gulping breath.

A prolapsed, or fallen, cord is serious business. The umbilical cord, the pulsing red lifeline that joins the baby and the mother and that supplies the baby with blood and oxygen, is normally tucked up at the top of the uterus beneath the baby's feet. And it stays there until the baby emerges, headfirst, from the womb, at which point the cord, attached at the baby's belly button, uncoils gradually, in response to the movement of the emerging infant through the birth canal. It's important that the cord remain safely coiled up in the top portion of the uterus while the baby is still in the womb, for each time the uterus contracts the cord is squeezed, slowing the flow of blood and oxygen. The upper portion of the uterus is roomy enough so that the cord isn't compressed too tightly, and there's still a sufficient supply of blood and oxygen, even during the fiercest contractions. But sometimes the cord falls into the lower portion of the uterus, which is already crowded with the baby's body. In severe cases, the slippery loops of coil will fall below the baby's head, through the narrow opening of the womb, out into the vagina. Then the uterus, contracting like a clenched fist, crushes the cord between the baby's head and the contracting wall of the uterus, completely cutting off the baby's supply of blood and oxygen. Such babies have to be delivered by cesarean section, and it must be done quickly.

"Well," I said, doubtful of his diagnosis, "let's take a look," and I went into the room. The woman was lying on the examining room table, her feet up in stirrups.

"The baby's coming!" she cried, grabbing both my hands in hers as I came up beside her.

"It's all right," I told her in my hearty, everything-is-under-control, doctor's voice. "I'm just going to take a look at you and see what's going on here."

I reached my gloved hand up inside her vagina. Everything was not under control. I could feel several loops of slippery coil. Almost the entire length of the cord had prolapsed into the vagina. I quickly explained to the woman that there was a problem and that we were going to have to take the baby by cesarean. While I was explaining, she began having a contraction. I pushed the cord back up into the uterus and held the baby's head against the front wall of the uterus in order to reduce the pressure on the cord as much as possible. Howie wheeled the gurney out of the room and down the hall as I ran alongside, my hand still in the woman's uterus.

"You're doing fine, just fine," I told her, "but when you feel the next contraction, I want you to resist the urge to push. Okay? Don't push. Now, remember, don't push."

By this time, the woman, thoroughly terrified, had lapsed into Spanish, her native tongue. She couldn't understand anything I was saying. I repeated the few Spanish words I knew.

"No empuje. No empuje. ¿Entiende? No empuje." (Don't push, don't push.)

"Si, doctor, si," she agreed softly.

We burst through the doors of the delivery room, the metal frame of the gurney clattering and clanging over the threshold. I felt the uterus begin to tighten again, drawing in on itself, and I braced myself. The force of a contracting uterus is incredibly powerful. It was like having my hand slammed in a car door. I bit my lip to keep from crying out.

The anesthesiologist was ready, needle poised. He slid the IV into the woman's arm as we transferred her to the delivery table. One of the staff doctors had scrubbed and was ready to take over. My hand was so numb, I couldn't have operated. The nurse poured antiseptic over the abdomen. The staff doctor pulled the steel blade across her belly, spreading the bloody wound to reveal the rosy, swollen uterus. We clamped and suctioned quickly, staying the flow of blood. Deftly, holding the knife lightly in his fingertips, as one holds a fiddle bow, he drew a short, sharp stroke, opening a small incision in the uterus. He angled the blunt snout of the surgical scissors into the incision, quickly enlarging the opening. Dropping the scissors onto the waiting tray, his hand groped through the enlarged incision into the womb, feeling for the baby's head. He palmed the baby's face in one hand, and with the other hand pressing on the top of the uterus, he pushed and pulled the baby out of the womb. We held our breath as he lifted the chalky white, toneless body out of her belly. The baby wasn't breathing. The surgeon barked orders, and we went through the rituals of revival, trying to breathe life back into the small, limp body; but it was no good. The cord had been crushed in too many places and circulation stopped for too long a time. The baby was dead.

We'd done all that was humanly possible, but the prolapse had been too severe. There was no way we could have saved the baby. It had been a goner before the woman ever got to us. Even if we'd done the c-section on the front steps of the hospital, we would still have lost the baby.

Howie and I worked in silence, closing up the abdominal incision. Howie fumbled, cutting the sutures too short.

"Too short," I told him, and maybe I should have said something more, something about what had just happened, but there wasn't anything more to say. It happens that way sometimes. You lose some. That's the way it goes. If Howie wanted to practice medicine, he'd have to learn to accept that. Besides, I didn't have time to say anything. I was being paged again.

This time, it was the head nurse from the labor suite calling to tell me that she thought Norma Thomas, one of the women in labor, was about to deliver. I was surprised. She'd been in labor only a couple of hours, and the last time I'd checked her, she'd still had a ways to go. I knew better than to doubt an experienced labor and delivery nurse, though. When you're a medical student or an intern, just starting out in this business of birthing, the L&D nurses, the kindhearted ones, take you aside and whisper advice:

"She has that look about the eyes, and her cries are turning to grunts—she's ready to go."

Or, "See those beads of sweat on her forehead? When they get like that, you've got to get them over to Delivery real quick."

You're full of your fancy medical school education and smug with scientific certainties about degrees of effacement and centimeters of dilation and other medical jabberwocky. You smile at their old wives' tales. Condescension dripping from your lips, you inform the nurse that this woman is only seven centimeters dilated and she's not even fully effaced; it will be hours before she delivers. Ten minutes later, the woman delivers right in her bed because you didn't get her over to Delivery in time. You don't make an ass of yourself in that particular way too many times.

Besides, I wanted to be sure Norma was fully anesthetized before hard labor began. I'd seen her in the OB clinic for one of her prenatal visits, and she'd been adamant about anesthesia, which wasn't what I expected. Norma was a nurse, and most nurses, the young ones anyhow, were devotees of the then new Lamaze method of natural childbirth. Not Norma. But then Norma was not the expected sort. She worked in the cardiac intensive care unit. She was an excellent nurse, and patients adored her. She was sassy and brassy and funny and a bit outrageous. Somehow that combination allowed her to skate right past the usual doctor-nurse politics. I'd never met her before I saw her in the OB clinic, but her reputation had preceded her. The stories about her were legion. It was said that she'd even stopped the temperamental star surgeon of the cardiac unit right in the middle of one of his instrument-flinging, operating room tantrums, and told him that if he didn't stop yelling and carrying on, she and the rest of the scrub nurses were taking a walk and he could operate by his damn self.

I only half believed all this until I finally met her,

when she came into OB clinic for one of her prenatal visits. She was not one of those nice, sweet ladies in gingham dresses who sit docilely across the desk and listen obediently to doctor's orders.

"Look," she told me, "in case you're on call the night I deliver—and I will deliver at night, women in my family always deliver smack in the middle of the night—I want you to know something. I want the whole works. I don't want to feel a thing. I let those lying Lamaze witches talk me into natural childbirth the first time. They said it wouldn't hurt, which is a bold-faced lie. It hurt like hell. So, if you're on that night, you be sure and remember that this lady gets everything you got to give her."

I told her I'd be sure to remember that, hoping I wouldn't be on duty the night she delivered. I was sure she'd insist on being scoped. Being scoped meant getting a drug called scopolamine. Actually, scopolamine wasn't even a painkiller; but it made the patients groggy and produced an amnesia deep enough that they didn't remember the pain afterwards, which is what made women think it was a wonderful painkiller. For some reason I no longer recall, being scoped also meant getting additional drugs. The combination made most women so incoherent that they couldn't organize themselves enough to scream during labor; that feature made it popular with doctors and L&D nurses too. But at this point in time, 1967, we didn't use it very much anymore, because we'd discovered there were some complications associated with the scopolamine regime. The scopolamine was administered by injection, in combination with a drug-impregnated mask which was placed over the woman's nose and mouth. The drugs in the mask would vaporize, the woman would inhale the fumes, and when she'd inhaled enough, her head would loll sideways and the mask would fall off. When she came 'round again, she'd grope for the mask, get it back on her face and grog out again. The complications, as we euphemistically called them, arose when a couple of women's heads failed to loll sideways and they OD'd. (Science marches on.) So, we didn't use the scopolamine and anesthesia mask anymore unless someone could be with the woman the entire time—and that just wasn't practical on a busy OB ward. But I doubted practicalities would matter much to Norma if she decided that scopolamine was the drug for her.

The other problem with the drug was that it sent some women right out into the ozone. They'd get fist-flailingly violent or suddenly get some strange notion in their heads. One woman, scoped to the gills, decided on the delivery table that, on second thought, she really didn't want a baby after all, so she might as well go on home. The baby was already halfway out of her, but she loped, bowlegged, all the way down the hall and was actually in the elevator before we caught up with her.

Having done battle with enough scoped women and having collected enough black eyes, I'd developed Patterson's Law of Scopolamine: Thou shall not be scoped while Patterson is on duty unless thou art smaller than Patterson. Since there aren't many full-term pregnant women who weigh less than a hundred and five, there weren't very many who qualified. Norma, who was five ten and hefty, definitely wasn't a candidate.

"All I've had is a shot of Demerol," she complained as I came in the room. "Scope me. I'm hurting."

"I'll do you one better," I told her after I examined her. "I'll take you over to Delivery and the anesthesiologist."

"Well, get a move on. Get me over there and knock me out," she demanded. I could see that despite her bluster, Norma really was uncomfortable, and more than a little afraid.

As it turned out, it was just as well that Norma had chosen to be fully anesthetized. The delivery itself was routine, but as soon as I saw the back of the baby's head, I knew something was very wrong. There weren't any skull bones. The baby was anencephalic, a condition in which there is only a minimal amount of brain tissue and a total lack of skull bones. Although the facial bones of an anencephalic develop properly, the lack of skull bones grossly distorts the face, giving it a grotesque, froglike appearance. The baby was born dead, and it wasn't a pretty sight. I was glad Norma didn't have to see it.

Running completely on automatic, I finished up in Delivery and went over to the doctor's lounge to get a cup of coffee, have a cigarette and pull myself together. My nerves were shot. Obstetrical deaths are a rarity, and two in a row virtually unheard of. I stuck a cigarette in my mouth backwards and lit the filter. Sputtering and coughing, I looked anxiously around the room, but no one else was there. I was afraid someone might have seen my fumbling with the cigarette, and then they would have known how unnerved I was. I couldn't let that happen. A doctor has to be tough. You can't let things get to you, or you won't be able to do your job properly. You can't get emotional about things. You have to maintain control. Doctors are in the business of controlling, or at least trying to control, the course of life and death. The neat, ordered little world of rules and regulations, starched white linen and stainless steel, with which we attempt to defy the messy mysteries of life and death, is fragile at best. If we were to start getting emotional, it could all come tumbling down. No, we couldn't let our emotions get out of hand. We had to keep a tight rein.

Because I was a woman, it was especially important that no one suspect, not even for a second, that I was at all shaken. Women, you see, are naturally suspect. As everyone in the medical profession knows, women are terribly emotional and not very good at controlling their emotions. All through medical school I heard stories about women doctors who "just weren't tough enough," who "just couldn't take it," who "broke down," who "fell apart." (I envisioned a great slag heap where broken-down women doctors, their limbs all akimbo, were stacked in huge mounds that reached the sky.) I had to prove that I was different.

I'd vowed to be as tough, as unemotional, as professional, as any of my male colleagues. And on the outside I was. No one ever saw me cry. But on the inside it was another story. They were, of course, entirely right about women doctors. I knew, because I knew how it was inside me.

Inside me there was a lone woman in long robes, standing at the edge of a darkened lake, wringing her hands in sorrow and weeping in despair. The Lady never did anything. She just stood there crying. I had no use for her and would like to have been rid of her. I never knew but that I'd forget for a moment to keep her quiet and she would cry loud enough to attract attention to herself and then someone might look at me and see her there. Because of her, I lived in constant fear of being found out.

I was disgusted with her, too. A simple fool with a bad attitude, she was an embarrassment to me, standing around, moping and whining all the time. Did she think she was ever going to get anywhere that way? I was furious with her. I wanted to get on about my business, but there she was with her tears.

I lit another cigarette. The truth was that I was having a hard time keeping her quiet because I could feel her tears move in me and taste her grief in my mouth. Because the world is much too sad a place for any of us to live in. Because two babies had just died in my arms. Because two lives were over before they'd be-

gun. Because I'd failed, and the failure stung as hard
as the grief.

Perhaps that sounds strange. It *is* strange, but for
doctors, death means more than the normal feelings
of grief and loss. Somewhere in our fantasies of ourselves, death is the enemy against which the Great
White Doctor battles. When death wins, the doctor
has lost, and doctors, perhaps more than most people, don't like to lose; death is a personal affront. I
have even known doctors to become angry with their
patients for dying. I wasn't that far gone, but some of
the Lady's tears were shed in self-pity at my failure.

So I sat there then, full of grief and loss and sad-
ness, and it was all mixed up with this sense of failure
and despair. The Lady was crying louder and louder,
and any minute now someone was going to hear her,
so I did what I had to do. I made her shut up. I had to.

Then, less than two hours later, I was back in the
delivery room. I knew Sheila Hart, the woman who
was about to give birth. She and her husband, Peter,
had recently returned from the Peace Corps, and I'd
seen them throughout the course of the pregnancy.
They were young and bright and well educated and
could have written their tickets anywhere. Instead,
they'd gone off to some impoverished corner of the
planet and had come back now, their idealism tested
and true, full of wonderful, warm stories, without
sounding like missionaries. They made you think that
everything was possible.

They'd taken natural childbirth classes, and their
excitement and enthusiasm about the birth was conta-
gious. Her labor had been relatively easy. She was in
some pain, but with the breathing exercises and her
husband's coaching, she was managing just fine. I
was glad it had turned out that they would deliver on
my shift. The delivery was going smoothly, which I
needed after the two previous deliveries.

The baby's head was crowning, and I told the

mother to go ahead and push with the next contraction. She gave a low grunt and bore down. The baby's head emerged, face down, and turned slowly to the side as the shoulder rotated under the pubic bone. She grunted more forcefully and pushed harder with the next contraction. The baby's upper shoulder came free. I arranged the receiving blanket in my lap, and waited for the next contraction, which I suspected would push most or all of the baby's body out of the birth canal. She grunted lower and deeper than before, and as the contraction reached its peak, I elevated the baby's head and applied a gentle downward traction. Sure enough, the entire body emerged.

Or what there was of it. It had no legs or feet. The body below the diaphragm muscle had not formed properly; instead, there was a thin, saclike structure where the baby's torso should have been. I could see the barely functioning internal organs through the transparent membrane of the sac. Horror-struck, I gingerly lowered the body to my lap. Everyone in the room froze. Somehow I managed, in a strangled voice, to tell the parents that the baby was deformed and that I didn't want them to see it.

I just sat there then, staring at the thing in my lap, watching as life slowly flowed out of it. The diaphragm muscles couldn't contract, so the baby couldn't breath. It strangled to death in my lap. I was paralyzed with shock and afraid to move, as I knew that the slightest movement might tear the skin of the sac, spilling the baby's entrails all over my lap.

Fortunately, the nurses took over. One turned her attention to the mother and father. Another covered the bottom half of the baby's body with a blanket. Someone had apparently called the chief, while I sat there, dumb with grief. I felt a gentle pressure on my shoulder. The chief laid a hand on my shoulder and said, "Doctor, why don't you let me take over here. Go on out to the lounge and take a break."

He reached over and lifted the dead baby out of my lap. The sac broke, and the baby's blood splashed into my lap. I just sat there staring helplessly at the blood. One of the nurses took me by the elbow and led me out of the delivery room. She sat me down in the lounge and lit a cigarette for me. I inhaled deeply and started crying, choking on my tears and the smoke.

I don't know how long I sat there crying—a long time, I think. The Lady of the Lake was on the loose, and hers was no longer a subdued, despairing weeping. These were not appealing fair-damsel-in-distress tears, the ones that melt hearts and make people want to take care of you. This was naked, madwoman-howling-at-the-moon, air-gulping, honking, red-faced sobbing, the kind that makes everyone want to leave the room. So I sat there alone, and cried and cried and cried. I was making a spectacle of myself, and I had it on strictest authority (from my mother) that making a public spectacle of yourself was about the most thoroughly disgraceful thing a woman could do. But the Lady of the Lake had never met my mother.

I'd lived with fear for such a long time: fear of public spectacles, fear of breaking down, fear of not being tough enough, fear of "acting like a woman," fear of failure, fear of death, fear of my inadequacy in the face of death, fear of my own death, fear of fear. Fear is a fussy houseguest. It moves in and starts rearranging all your things, and pretty soon you can't find yourself anymore. But for the moment I'd let go of the lease that fear had on me. I just didn't care about being tough or controlled or professional. And somewhere in the midst of all this, it began to seem utterly absurd that I should be sitting there crying by myself until I could pull myself together enough to go out and see the parents.

For one thing, that might have taken forever. For another, I wanted to be with the people who would share at least some of what I was feeling. I was tired of crying alone in secret corners.

With tears still streaming down my face, and not caring who saw them, I made my way down the corridor to Sheila Hart's room. The three of us held each other and cried together. I don't know what we said. When the tears subsided enough, I tried to answer their questions. Why had it happened? I didn't know. Maybe it was all the immunization shots they'd had in the Peace Corps? No, I reassured them, it wasn't anything they'd done wrong, and it wasn't likely to happen again. I spent almost an hour with them. When I left, I left feeling cleansed. Despite the grief, I felt good. Something that had been frozen up inside me for a long time was beginning to thaw.

TWO

I DREAMT that night of fetuses, hundreds of them. The fetuses and I were on a sailboat way out in the middle of nowhere. They were at that four- or five-month stage, half formed but vaguely humanoid. They were not, however, the diagrammatic, immobile, womb-bound figures pictured in anatomy textbooks. These were charming, cherub-bellied creatures with chubby little arms and legs. They scurried to and fro, scrambling playfully about the decks, swinging from the mast and rolling and tumbling over each other like a litter of pups with no regard for their own safety, so that every now and again one would tumble overboard into the sea. But this was no problem, none at all, because Big Mama Me was there to scoop them out of the sea and lift them back to the safety of the deck. This was my job, and in my dream I was good at it.

It was a sunny, sea-bright day, and everything was floating and anxiety-free and really quite pleasant until, as sometimes happens in dreams, the weather was suddenly all turned around. Day turned to night, and we sailed on a grave sea under an ominous green moon. I reached overboard after one of the fetuses, but it slipped from my grasp and slid beneath the surface of the sea. I dove in after it.

The sea was thick like Jell-O, and I could hardly swim through it. I struggled toward the tiny body which kept appearing and disappearing in the grey-

19

green depths. I sensed the huge vastness of the sea around me, and felt in contrast as tiny as the fetus. Still, I swam after it. But it was so distant and so far away and so hard to reach that the harder I struggled, the more distant it became.

I woke still reaching for it, chased out of my sleep by my dream and by those terrible feelings of guilt and failure and helplessness that had been born out of the death of the three babies. I lingered for a moment in that strange limbo between sleep and wakefulness, unable to get free of the dream and reluctant to move into full waking consciousness.

I woke with the peculiar sort of disorientation we feel when we wake in a strange place, so that at first I wasn't sure where I was. Then the dream slid away. The familiar on-call room took shape around me. The events of the night before came flooding in on me, and all I wanted was to curl up in a ball and pull the covers over my head or crawl under the bed and hide. I was ashamed, embarrassed at myself and mortified by the way I'd behaved, and all I could hear were these voices inside my head. They were prim, punishing voices, and they went on and on about public spectacles and disgraceful displays of emotion and how could I have been so unprofessional, and they drowned out everything else. The release I'd felt the night before was gone, and all I had left was the memory of having fallen apart, of having broken down, of having acted like all those women doctors whom I had been warned about. I was like a guilty drunk on the morning after a hazy night before, who can't exactly remember what was done or said on a boozy breath, but knows with a terrible certainty that it was something unforgivable. Whatever it was inside me that had started to thaw that night had frozen right back up again, just like that, and to this day I'm not sure how it happened so quickly.

Maybe it was the dream; but I doubt it was that

alone that made me wake up so far away from what I'd felt the night before. I think the same thing would have happened, dream or no, because changing, coming to a new place within oneself, is not an easy presto-and-it's-done kind of thing. It's not as simple as the pop psychologies make it sound when they promise to rearrange and reframe your psyche in one jargon-filled weekend session. It's not as easy as the born-agains, with their miraculous repentances and instantaneous conversions, find it.

I can never quite accept those Moment-of-Truth-That-Changed-My-Life stories. There are too many moments of truth in a lifetime, and as far as I can tell, personal change, enduring and transforming change, is never such a quick piece of business. At least for me, it has always been a much more time-consuming and dragged out affair.

The problem with those Moment of Truth stories is that they never tell you anything about the moments after the moment of truth. Revelations, epiphanies and peak experiences are all very fine, but we aren't Olympic gods to go leaping from peak to peak; between those mountaintops lie deep and yawning valleys and many flat plains.

This business of change is never so straightforward as the pop psychologists, the born again, and the Moment-of-Truthers make it seem. It's almost always a two-steps-backward/one-step-forward kind of process. I suspect there is a psychic law in the universe akin to the physical law that says: For every action, there is an equal and opposite reaction, so that changing is a process of opening up and closing back down, of grandly taking risks and then reactively clutching at security, of moving forward and then sliding back. I guess what I'm trying to say here is that maybe the best we can hope for when the winds of change blow us down is enough of a bounce on the rebound so that ultimately we land a little farther along than we were when we started. That's something, and maybe even enough to get by on.

At any rate, I did not wake up the next morning defrosted and healthy and whole, and I did not live happily ever after. This is not that easy a story. I moved forward that night, but by the next morning I had slid way back.

I lay there in my bed in the on-call room that morning, utterly miserable and all ragged around the edges, having trouble remembering exactly what had happened. It was all so hazy. I remembered this . . . this *creature* being born. I had lowered it into my lap; and then what? I'd been paralyzed for a time by the shock of it all. The next thing I clearly remembered was the chief being there and lifting the tiny body out of my lap, and all that blood everywhere.

The blood . . . the blood had been the baby's blood. The mother wasn't hemorrhaging, was she? She couldn't have been. I wouldn't have just sat there staring at the blood if the mother had been bleeding, if she had needed medical attention. Would I have? Could I have?

Someone *had* called for the chief, though. . . . I tried to tell myself that they almost always paged for a staff doctor when a baby delivered by a resident was stillborn. But I couldn't quite convince myself. Right on the nagging edge of my mind was the terrible thought that I'd blown it, that I'd been in such a state of shock I'd been unable to function and that was why they'd called for someone else.

I had a sudden, sickening feeling that that was what had happened. I hadn't been able to function. One of the nurses had seen that and she'd paged for help. The chief had responded to the page, and when *he* saw that I was unable to function, he'd told me I could go on out to the lounge because it was obvious that I wouldn't be of any use in the situation.

All I could remember after that was the crying. The Lady of the Lake had taken over, and, oh God, had the chief seen me like that? I was trying to remember. I didn't think so. I didn't think I'd started crying until I went out into the lounge. But I wasn't sure. I simply wasn't sure about any of it. I didn't know how long I'd sat there, paralyzed with shock. I didn't know why he'd sent me out of the room. I didn't know whether he'd seen me crying. I didn't know, so of course I assumed the worst.

If the worst was true, if I'd blown it in the delivery room and someone else had had to take over, then what would happen? Well, it would be bad, very bad. The chief would call me into his office. Oh, he'd be very nice about it, but he'd have no choice really, he'd have to let me go. You couldn't afford to have doctors in the delivery room or in OR who fell apart under pressure. Maybe he'd offer to help me find a place in another residency program. Probably he would. No one wants to see all those years of medical training go down the tubes. Maybe he'd suggest that I consider another speciality—something like pathology, where you weren't involved in patient care, where you couldn't blow it when the pressure was on. Or maybe he'd find me something in medical research, something in the basement of the hospital, in the rat labs, where I wouldn't be a danger to patients.

It was still early. My alarm hadn't even gone off yet, but I decided to get dressed and go on down to the staff cafeteria and eat breakfast before anyone else got there. I wasn't ready to face anyone yet.

I went through the cafeteria line, taking only two slices of wilted toast and a cup of black coffee. The cafeteria was empty except for a couple of residents from another service—and the very person I least wanted to see.

The chief saw me before I could drop my tray and run, which was my first impulse. "Jane!" His big voice boomed across the empty room at me. "Just the person I was looking for. Bring your tray over here."

Clutching my tray with both hands as though it might hold me up, I made my way stiff-legged across the cafeteria, and managed to sink into a chair across the table from him.

"My god," he said, looking at my lone plate of toast. His tray was heaped with half-eaten food— eggs, sausages, pancakes, bacon, donuts, juice, milk, coffee. "Is that all you eat for breakfast?" He shook his head. "Well, it's no wonder."

"No wonder what?" I squeaked. It was a dumb thing to say, but it was the thought in my head, and out it came. I was expecting the worst—no wonder I was such a lousy doctor, no wonder I couldn't function properly, no wonder he was going to have to fire me.

"No wonder you're such a tiny little thing. You should eat more. Here," he said through a muffled mouthful of eggs, "have some pancakes." And he pushed the plate onto my tray.

Obediently I took a bite of pancake.

"I've been wanting to talk to you about next year," he said, still eating.

I tried to swallow the doughy wad of pancake in my mouth, but it wouldn't go past the lump in my throat.

"You know that I had originally scheduled you for the first three-month rotation on regular OB, but last night I realized that I needed to make some changes in the schedule for next year."

This was it. Now it was coming. My mouth was dry. The pancake was still lodged in my throat and I couldn't say anything. I just nodded at him.

"I'd like to put you on complicated OB first, but I see that you requested your vacation in the beginning of the year, and I like to have the senior resident on comp OB there the whole time. How would you feel about taking your vacation later in the year?"

I swallowed the pancake. "Complicated OB?" My voice wasn't quite so squeaky. "Next year?" I said. "You want me next year, this next year coming up you want me to—" I was double-checking, still not quite believing what I was hearing.

"I want you to take your vacation later in the year, Jane," he interrupted me, sounding slightly annoyed. "Of course, if you've made some specific vacation plans, if there's something more important to you than—"

"Oh no, sir, no. I didn't have any plans for next year, none at all."

"Well, good, then," he said, "that's settled. Here, have a donut. I'm not very hungry." This was hardly surprising, since he'd cleaned off almost his entire tray. "Don't have my usual appetite this morning," he explained. "I was up all night. Just as I was leaving last night, a woman came into ER with lower abdominal pains. They thought maybe it was appendicitis, but they wanted to get a gynecology consult. I happened to be there, so I took a look. You won't believe what it turned out to be—a bilateral ectopic pregnancy."

Even in my befuddled state, I could appreciate his amazement. An ectopic pregnancy occurs when the fertilized egg doesn't make it down to the uterus, and implants instead in one of the fallopian tubes. An ectopic can be a life-threatening situation, because the tube is too small to accommodate the growing pregnancy. The tube may burst and the woman will start bleeding internally, and may even die. Ectopic pregnancies are not all that uncommon, but a *bilateral* ectopic pregnancy is a different story. It involves two ectopic pregnancies, one in each tube—a twin ectopic pregnancy. They are extremely rare.

"When we opened her up, there was so much pressure in the abdomen that the blood hit the operating lights. It was pretty touch and go for a while, but she's going to make it. Anyway, I was up all night with her. Oh, but that's right," he said, "you were here too, weren't you? I'd forgotten. That was a hard one, wasn't it? Nice couple, too. Hart, isn't that their name? Bizarre case. I guess it was just that kind of night. Be sure to show me the pathology report on that when it comes back, will you? I don't suppose it will tell us much, though—never does with these unusual deformities. Well, see you on rounds at nine. Eat up now." And with that, he pushed his bulk away from the table and made his way out of the cafeteria, leaving me sitting there, all weak in the knees.

So it was okay. They weren't going to banish me to the basement. I wouldn't have to spend the rest of my life peering into a microscope or chasing rats around the hospital lab. I hadn't blown it in a crisis situation. They'd paged for someone only because it was routine procedure to page a staff doctor if a resident was handling a case and the baby was stillborn. The chief had just happened to be in the area. He'd come in and taken over, not because I'd been incompetent, but because it was a messy case and it was late and that's the kind of guy he was.

It was all a lot clearer to me now. The nurse had lit a cigarette for me, and then she'd left me alone there crying. Maybe she'd seen me crying, but the chief and staff doctors hadn't, and that was the important thing. I'd gone down to Sheila Hart's room, and I'd still been pretty upset at that point, but it was so late at night there couldn't have been anyone else on the ward besides the night nurse, and it didn't really matter that much if she'd seen me like that.

So I hadn't been found out. I was going to get away with it. I sat there toying with the food on the tray. I'd been lucky; I hadn't gotten caught. But those prim, punishing voices started in again. My behavior had been inexcusable, totally unprofessional. That was what came from getting too personal with your patients. Good doctors don't do that. I vowed then and there that I would never, never do that again.

It had never been too difficult for me to maintain the proper sort of emotional distance with patients before. I am by nature a shy person, and I grew up in a family where emotional contact was sparse. My parents were nice people who were concerned about my welfare, who made sure that my socks were on straight and that I ate everything on my plate. But they both came from rigid, Scotch Protestant backgrounds, and were not the sort of people into whose arms you'd fling yourself, sobbing passionately when your puppy dog died or some other childhood tragedy struck you down cold in the middle of your hopscotch game. They couldn't understand the trauma of not being invited to someone's birthday party or the triumph of losing both your front teeth on the same day. Skinned knees were treated sensibly with Mercurochrome and Band-Aids, not with hugs and kisses. They were good people, but rather aloof and remote. They just didn't have the emotional equipment for responding to a child's triumphs, traumas and tragedies. We were not a family given to spontaneous displays of emotionality, and I developed the habit of keeping my feelings to myself. Establishing emotional contact was not something I did with any ease or facility.

My medical training did nothing to change that. Contact with patients during medical school and internship is fleeting. The patients come into the hospital, you take care of them, they go home, and you never see them again. You're always rotating to different hospitals or different wards, so you never really get to know anyone very well. For most doctors, it's the same during the residency.

The hospital where I worked was a little different, though. It was the major medical facility for the members of a prepaid medical insurance plan. Individual members and their employers paid a monthly fee that covered all medical expenses, so we saw many of the same people regularly. I might operate on a woman and then see her a few weeks later in the clinic for her post-op checkup, and maybe I'd see her again a few months later in OB clinic for a prenatal visit. I might even be on duty the night she delivered. Patients were beginning to be recognizable individuals. Even so, it was unusual that I got to know anyone as well as I knew the Harts. We residents were always being transferred from one ward to another so that we'd have an opportunity to gain experience in all the different aspects of our speciality. It was rare that I would actually happen to be working in the OB clinic each time a certain woman came in for her prenatal visits, and rarer still that I would happen to be on call and would end up delivering her baby.

Also, there's a peculiar thing that happens to doctors during training; I don't exactly know how to explain it. We start out, our heads crammed full of all these idealistic notions about alleviating human suffering and stamping out disease. For me it was a combination of Ben Casey and Florence Nightingale with a dash of white-knight-in-shining-armour thrown in. And then we find ourselves surrounded by sick people and piss and shit and vomit, and none of it is the least bit noble. Interns and residents are terribly overworked and never have enough sleep. Somehow it turns into a them-against-us proposition and the patients to whom you were going to be such a dandy Florence Nightingale end up being the enemy.

I think it really started to get to me when I was assigned to the acute medicine ward at the VA hospital as an intern. "Acute medicine"—it had such a dramatic ring to it. I had visions of racing about in my white coat saving lives. The acute medicine ward at the VA hospital turned out to be a drunk tank. Most of the beds were taken up by alcoholics. A lot of them lived there at the VA hospital in a special housing project, a sort of concentration camp for diseased veterans, called the Domicilary. These men would get their monthly disability checks and trot over to the aptly named Windfall, a bar across the street, and get falling down drunk and be brought back across the street to the hospital. When they came to, they'd have the DT's, so there would be this forty-bed ward of raving lunatics screaming about the snakes or bugs that were after them. We used to treat the DT's with a drug called paraldehyde, which they didn't like to take. So there I'd be at three o'clock in the morning with some raving lunatic old gomer screaming, ''Get away from me you evil hunched-over whore dog'' and spitting paraldehyde in my face and vomiting cheap, sour booze all over me.

The whole place looked like something out of Marat/Sade, and smelled like urine, because after a while the patients' diseased livers couldn't process the ammonia out of their bodies anymore. In the later stages of alcoholism, the blood vessels in the esophagus go and the patients begin vomiting up blood. So I'd have to get up in the middle of the night—and it always was the middle of the night—to stop the bleeding, which was done by inserting a tube with balloon-like attachments down their throats. That done, I'd inflate the balloons and hope this would put enough pressure on the blood vessels to stop the bleeding. The drunks didn't like having things stuck down their throats, and they thrashed and swung at their would-be saviours, shouting obscenities and vomiting blood the whole time. In a day or two, they'd check out of the hospital against medical advice and go get drunk again. And then those of us who'd been on duty would get chewed out for not keeping them in the hospital because the VA hospital budget was determined by bed occupancy percentage. The more beds occupied for the longer time, the higher the budget allocation, so we were supposed to keep someone until we had another body to take his place. Maybe it wouldn't have been quite so bad, maybe we could have pretended that all the vomit and blood soaking through our clothes right down to our underwear at some ungodly hour of the morning was worth it because a life was being saved, except that in a week or a month the same old gomer would be back again, vomiting blood and screaming obscenities as a tube was being stuffed down his throat. It didn't feel a bit like Ben Casey or Florence Nightingale.

Or maybe it started even before that disastrous three months on the acute medicine ward at the VA. My first rotation as an intern had been on the gynecology ward at the university hospital. It wasn't a typical gynecology ward. Almost all the patients had advanced cancer. They'd usually been treated elsewhere in the early stages and had been transferred to the university hospital as a last resort so we could try out on them whatever new form of medication we were experimentally pumping into veins to try to halt the spread of cancer. Or if the women weren't getting medication, they were in for some radical form of cancer surgery. Their insides were taken out, so they had bags to shit in and bags to urinate in and tubes to eat through and were at best semicomatose. But we were bent on saving their lives, so when their hearts stopped beating and their lungs gave out, we rushed in and pumped their hearts and pushed air into their lungs because it was our job to keep them alive. And I had my doubts. I'd tell myself that this one seemed a little better, a little perkier than last week, so maybe it was okay to pound on her chest and get her heart back into action to keep her alive for a little while longer. Maybe the family hovering around her bedside still had things to say, things to finish with her. Maybe that extra week of life we forced back into the dying body provided a few lucid moments when things could be said between the dying woman and her loved ones that would bring some sort of necessary closure. Who was I to know these unfathomable things? And besides, I was learning how to perform all those miracles of bringing someone back to life, skills that I might be able to use someday to save someone who wasn't irretrievably dying of cancer, someone who, if she or he could be brought through a crisis, might go on to live a normal, healthy life. So maybe it was okay to pump life back into someone who would then have another incredibly painful week of living death to endure; but it got hard to believe that when patients would grab my hands and beg me to leave them alone and let them die in peace.

I didn't know what to do or say or how to behave with a dying person. This wasn't included in medical school curriculums in my day. These women were dying, and I was terrified of their deaths. They were dying of gynecological cancers, and I was a woman, and maybe I would die like that. My terror of their deaths was all entwined with my terror of my own death. I kept my distance.

My internship rotations in surgery, pediatrics and obstetrics weren't quite so macabre, but patient contact was fleeting and the habit of keeping my distance was by then a well-ingrained survival mechanism. Besides, we were so overworked and underslept. The obstetrics ward was particularly hectic. I think I delivered over a hundred babies in one month. The place was a regular baby factory. Drug 'em up, wheel 'em in, pull out the baby, run to the next room and catch the next baby—a factory line operation. These weren't women, human beings, about to give birth; they were baby production units.

And they were out to get you. Like the drunks on the acute medicine ward—they were out to get you. As soon as you fell asleep, another one would come in. Cranky and overtired, you'd drag out of bed, grumbling and complaining and in a thorough purple funk because some woman had to have her goddamn baby at four-thirty in the morning. And you knew she did it on purpose, just to get you out of bed.

And so it was that, before my residency, maintaining the prescribed emotional distance with patients had never been a great problem for me. But my residency *was* different from my previous medical experience. I'd begun to relax my guard. But, I'd learned my lesson with the Harts!

Really though, it wasn't entirely my fault, I told myself as I sat there in the cafeteria, still searching for excuses. It was this natural childbirth business. When something like this happened, the parents were *right there*. If the mother had been anesthetized and if the father had been out in the waiting room where fathers were supposed to be, it wouldn't have happened the way it did. I could have spoken to the father in the waiting room and to the mother when she came to. It was the two of them being there, that stricken look on their faces, that made me lose control.

I needed a scapegoat, I needed to subtract myself from the situation, and natural childbirth was the perfect scapegoat. I sat there toying with my food, building up the case against natural childbirth. I had been leery of the whole business right from the first time I ran into it—and *ran into* is a very deliberate choice of words here, because it was a head-on collision.

It was just after I'd completed my internship, during the first month or so of my residency. I was on call in OB, and about two in the morning a nurse from Labor called, complaining about a woman who was refusing to let them start her IV. I was furious with the nurse for waking me, *the doctor*, in the middle of the night for something so trivial. Starting IV's was a nursing job.

"If you can't handle your patients, call your nursing supervisor, not me," I snapped, and hung up the phone, which immediately rang again.

"The nursing supervisor has already been called. The woman keeps refusing the IV and insists on seeing a doctor," she snapped right back, and hung up on me. (One of the things about being a woman doctor was that nurses took less shit from you than from the male doctors, which was a piece of salvation for me in the end, but which I saw as a lack of respect at the time.)

Thoroughly cranky, I muttered and grumbled my way down to Labor. This was going to be one of those women who bitch and moan and scream the whole way through their deliveries; I knew, just knew it. I was in one of those irrational snits that you can only work yourself into through a calculated program of sleep deprivation. I half hated the woman by the time I got to her room. But at the same time I was a bit curious about her. The L&D night nursing supervisor, Nurse McGowan, was a bulldog of a woman, an imposing figure; short, but massive and dense. She'd been an ambulance driver during World War II and had never quite lost the aura of the battlefield. She was formidable, and I couldn't imagine anyone not obeying her orders instantly.

"The nurse tells me there's some problem about your IV," I said with exaggerated, icy politeness. The woman turned her glazed eyes towards me. She was well into labor and obviously feeling it. She was tiny and pale, with delicate features and great masses of blond hair soaked with perspiration and sticking to her pillow. She looked like a worn-out angel. How had she managed to stand up to the Sherman tank approach that was the bedrock of the McGowan bedside manner? I started to soften towards her.

"We aren't having any IV's," announced a loud and belligerent voice behind my back. I turned around. It was the husband. I hadn't even noticed him when I came in the room—which said something about the state I was in. He was a hard guy to miss. He had even more hair than his wife and a wild beard. He wore patched and faded blue jeans, a Salvation Army Marching Band jacket, and had all manner of beads, feathers, and peace symbols dangling off him. This was, good lord, a hippie. Well, I knew all about hippies. I'd seen an article about them in *Life* magazine with full-color photos. They never cut their hair or took baths, and they smoked marijuana all the time.

I was probably the furthest possible thing from being a hippie, and we must have made an odd tableau, the two of us, standing there glaring at each other—he with his unkempt hair and his full-on, antiestablishment regalia; me with my hair pinned in a neat, precise bun atop my head, wearing my starched white doctor's uniform, the very embodiment of the middle-class establishment.

At any rate, the battle lines were drawn. He had met the establishment, and it was me. He had come prepared to do battle.

"We're not having any drugs, so you can forget about that. We're doing this our own way. This is going to be a natural childbirth. We're Lamaze trained," he said, as though that explained everything.

"You're La-what?" I said.

"Lamaze. Prepared childbirth. You're hip to Lamaze, right?" he said in a tone that implied that not having heard of Lamaze was like not having heard of sliced bread.

I just stood there looking blank.

"Well, dig, it's like this . . ." And he was off into a lingo-laden rap about "where he was coming from" and "where it was at" and "if I could dig it"—which I could not. None of it made a whit of sense to me, but I vaguely recalled having read an article somewhere or other about some group that was advocating child-birth without anesthesia. I had read the article and promptly dismissed it because it was such a ludicrous idea. It would set the practice of obstetrics back two hundred years, and why would anyone want to suffer pain when they didn't have to?

So, there I was with this creature, with roach clips dangling from his lapels and a packet of Zig-Zag papers in his pocket, lecturing me on how dangerous it was to use drugs, telling me what to do and what not to do in *my* labor room in *my* hospital. My feathers were more than a little ruffled. But I did not lose my temper: This person was obviously somewhat unbalanced, another California crazy. I had been out here from the East Coast long enough to recognize the type, and I knew how to deal with it. Adopting a tone I used with psychiatric patients and small children, I carefully explained that all I was going to do was to start an IV with some glucose in it.

"We don't want any drugs," he repeated, stubborn and hostile.

I explained that glucose was just sugar water, that his wife was in labor and that the sugar water would give her some energy and help her to keep her strength up.

"We wouldn't want her to get tired out, now would we?" I said, sounding like the lady on Romper Room.

"We brought these." He held up a plastic bag full of lollipops. "Natural barley sugar pops. If she needs energy, she can suck on these."

Terrific. Hippie with lollipops at two in the morning.

"Well, I'm afraid your wife can't have anything orally now that she's in labor," I began; but I could see that this was just going to get me more flack, so I switched tactics. "But, maybe, she could have one or two. So, now then, I'll just set up this IV and be out of your way. It will only take a few seconds."

"No IV," he said, folding his arms across his chest. "It'll interfere with her breathing."

Jesus, her breathing—what did he think I was going to do, stick it down her throat?

"Oh no, she'll be able to breathe just fine. I'm going to put the IV here in her hand," I said, reaching for the IV bottle.

"No way," he said, stepping between me and the IV bottle. "We aren't having any IV."

This was getting old, fast. "But the IV is a standard delivery room procedure." "Standard procedure" was for me an adequate explanation for anything. It had no impact whatsoever on him. "We need to have it started just in case your wife runs into problems and needs to be transfused—not that anything like that is likely to happen, but just in case. So, if you'll step aside here, I'll start this IV. It will just take a couple of seconds, and then I'll be out of here."

"Well," he insisted, not moving from in front of the IV, "if it takes only a couple of seconds, you can do it when and if she needs it."

We stood there glaring at each other, two gunslingers having it out at high noon, and might still be standing there, but his wife started having a contraction. He leapt to her side and propped her up in the bed.

"Now, remember, in through the nose and out through the mouth," he told her, and the two of them started breathing in unison, panting like two dogs in heat. It was easily the most peculiar piece of human behavior I'd ever seen.

"What . . . what . . ." I was trying to ask what they were doing, but the words wouldn't quite come out.

"Controlled breathing, for the pain," he said, turning to me after the contraction had passed.

Controlled breathing! I'd had enough. My patience was worn thin. These people were mad as hatters.

"That's all very nice, I'm sure, but I have other patients to see," I said through tight lips, making it sound as though there were whole wards of women awaiting my ministrations. "Do I understand that you're ignoring medical advice and are refusing the IV?"

He let me know once again that was exactly what he was doing, and made a rude anatomical suggestion about what I could do with the IV.

"Very well, then, I'll note your refusal on the chart, but I must tell you that the hospital cannot be held responsible if anything happens." And on that dire note, I swept out of the room.

Luckily for them, she didn't deliver until after I went off duty, not that they would have gotten any better treatment from the day staff. None of us was too open to Lamaze in those days.

This, then, had been my introduction to Lamaze. In the months that followed, more and more Lamaze couples had begun showing up in Labor and Delivery. We didn't exactly welcome them with open arms; we made fun of them behind their backs. One of the residents did what we considered to be a particularly hilarious imitation of a Lamaze mother panting and grunting her way through labor and delivery. If a Lamaze mother gave in and took the drugs we were always pushing at her, we walked around with triumphant smirks, feeling personally vindicated. In later years, when I became an unqualified Lamaze enthusiast, I told myself that our initial negative reaction and our reluctance to accept Lamaze was just part of the natural and justifiable conservatism of the medical profession. After all, one wouldn't want doctors jumping on the bandwagon of every new fad that comes along. But it ran much deeper than that. What Lamaze couples were saying was: Hey, this is not *your* turf. This is *our* birth, *our* experience, and we'll tell you how we want things to happen. The idea that the hospital should be run for the convenience or the emotional needs of the patients was an entirely radical notion. It ran counter to everything we had been trained to think about ourselves and our relative importance in the universe.

I don't remember exactly when it was that I was forced to notice the obvious, but somewhere along the line it began to dawn on me that the Lamaze mothers had shorter labors; that their undrugged babies were healthier, more alert; that they had easier deliveries. Even then, when these half-formed observations should have been obvious to me, I resisted the idea. My own sister, a nurse with two kids, had called me during this time: Did I think she should try Lamaze with her third pregnancy? Oh no, she shouldn't try it. She was a nurse, and there would be too much pressure on her. Even if she decided she wanted anesthesia, she might not ask for it, out of pride. Here you see the power of the medical mystique. Even my own sister, who had grown up with me and knew me for a fool, thought, because of the "MD" after my name, that my opinion had some magical authority. Despite my failure to respond to a single one of her questions about whether Lamaze would be better for the baby or her, she accepted my opinion completely.

Finally, after we'd been seeing Lamaze patients for months, the chief asked an RN who was a Lamaze coach to speak at one of our Thursday afternoon educational conferences. Maybe it was that she was an official person in white and that her talk was endorsed by the chief, but after that I began to realize not only that the labors were shorter and the babies healthier, but also that the mothers' attitudes towards their babies were much different. Under traditional L&D procedures the mothers remained groggy from the drugs for a day or so after giving birth, and when we brought the babies to them for the first time, many were listless and apathetic. The Lamaze mothers were bright-eyed and excited, cooing over their babies, delighted with themselves and the world. Maybe, just maybe, there was something to the whole thing.

Still, I remained wary of it. I couldn't quite analyze why at the time, but I think what made me uncomfortable was the fact that the Lamaze parents were right there in the delivery room and the mother wasn't drugged out. Suddenly it was no longer a matter of our doing something *to* a patient but of our working *with* the patient and her partner—a much more personal and involving process. Having to relate to patients as people was not something most doctors were prepared to do.

I sat there in the cafeteria that morning, sipping my coffee, with all these thoughts going through my head, letting all that leeriness sink back in. No doubt about it, this natural childbirth was bad business. Look what had happened to the Harts. By the time I'd finished my breakfast, I'd managed to work things around in my head so that the whole episode had very little to do with anything inside me or with the Lady of the Lake. It was all the fault of natural childbirth.

The one thing I was grateful for was that I wouldn't have to see the Harts again. I was working days on the GYN ward and was on call in OB only every fourth night. It would be three more nights before I'd be back in OB, and by then Sheila Hart would have been discharged.

Then I remembered: Sheila Hart had been transferred to GYN last night. I'd done it myself, not that it had been my idea to transfer her. As I was leaving the hospital the night before, one of the nurses had stopped and asked to talk to me. She was new on the floor, and I didn't know her very well. I was in no mood for casual chitchat, but I'd stopped to find out what she wanted.

"Uh, Dr. Patterson"—she was nervous about talking to me—"I know this isn't the way you usually do things around here, but at the hospital where I trained, we usually transferred the stillborns off the maternity ward. It's a lot easier for the mothers that way."

She was stepping outside the bounds, bypassing the normal channels of communication. The hospital is a hierarchical world. Nurses, especially the lower echelon ones, were not supposed to tell doctors what to do. If she had a suggestion about patient care, she should have talked to the head nurse, who would have passed it on to the staff doctor in charge of the floor if she thought it had merit. If he thought so too, he could have passed it on to me. But, what she was saying was so obviously the right thing to do. Mrs. Hart and the other two women didn't need to be on the OB ward with all the beatific new mothers and their bouncing babies, while they had only their grief to nurse. Besides, I was so slavishly grateful to be able to do something for these women that I forgot to summon up the frostiness the nurse's suggestions should have produced.

"Right, of course, I'll see what I can do," I told her. Gynecology hadn't been too happy about taking on three extra patients. They groused and grumbled, but in the end, they'd finally agreed to take them.

So, I now realized, I'd have to see the Harts, and I wanted to do it before rounds at nine o'clock. Everyone was there for rounds—the chief, the staff doctors, all the residents—and when we made rounds, we stopped at each patient's bedside to discuss the case. I wanted to see Sheila Hart alone first, without a whole crowd being there. It was going to be embarrassing enough as it was. I wasn't sure what I was going to say, but I decided it was better not to say anything about how I'd acted the night before. Best just to ignore it, pretend it had never happened. I'd be very professional, very matter of fact, and somehow I'd reestablish the proper sort of professional distance with her.

I stepped off the elevator onto the GYN ward, and there was Peter Hart.

"Oh, Dr. Patterson, I was hoping to see you." He looked like he'd been run over by something large and heavy. It was obvious from the stubble on his chin and his rumpled clothing that he'd spent the night at the hospital.

"Mr. Hart," I said, stiff and formal, "how are you? How is Mrs. Hart?"

"She's okay. I guess. You know. I think maybe she's sleeping. I don't know. They won't let me in to see her until visiting hours. I really appreciate your sending her over here instead of keeping her on the maternity ward, but there weren't any private rooms available over here, so they won't let me stay with Sheila, and I really want to be with her. Do you think I could go in and see her for just a few minutes at least?"

"Sure," I told him. "You go on in. I'll speak to the nurse. Just pull the curtain around the bed and keep your voice down so you don't disturb the other patients."

"Oh, and one other thing, Doctor," he said, "When do you think she can go home? I mean, is there really any reason for her to stay here? You've been great. Everyone's been great, but they keep trying to give her all these tranquilizers and sleeping pills and—"

"Well," I interrupted, "your wife's been through an ordeal. The sedatives will help to keep her calm." We routinely prescribed tranquilizers for women who had stillbirths. We told ourselves that they needed them.

"But the tranquilizers won't take away the pain. It would be better for us if we could just go home and do what we need to, make the funeral arrangements and all that, and just, well, just be together.''

I could see his point, and the idea of their being gone felt safer to me. I was probably as anxious to have them out of the hospital as they were to get out.

"I really don't see any reason why not, provided your wife isn't hemorrhaging or anything. I'll talk to your doctor and we'll discuss it when we see Mrs. Hart on rounds this morning."

"Thanks, thanks a lot, Dr. Patterson," he said, and went down the hall to his wife's room.

I spoke to the head nurse, explaining that I had given Peter Hart permission to be in his wife's room. She pursed her lips and clucked about how irregular it was and about established visiting hours and hospital routines being disrupted. I clucked right back at her, glad to have someone to take my anger out on.

I went down the hall to face Sheila Hart. I stood for a moment outside the door to her room. The curtains were drawn around the bed, but through a crack in the drapes, I could see the two of them. Peter was at her side, murmuring in a low voice, caressing her, gently pushing the hair away from her forehead in a rhythmic, soothing motion. I stood there watching them, transfixed by a sudden and overwhelming sense of loneliness.

I wasn't going in there. I wasn't going to risk myself in the middle of all that closeness. I wasn't doing that again.

As I was turning away, Sheila Hart spotted me through the crack in the drapes.

"Oh, Dr. Patterson," she called, "please come in."

So I had to.

"How are you, Mrs. Hart?" I asked in a voice I tried to make properly professional. I had already rehearsed what I would say to her, all those hearty condolences I had heard doctors use in these situations:

"You're young, you can try again."

"You'll be pregnant again before you know it."

"It was a blessing in disguise."

But all those lame platitudes just died on my lips before I could even bring the conversation around to them, because she took my hand and held it in hers and said, "Dr. Patterson, I want to thank you very much. You don't know how much we appreciated your being there like that with us last night. I can't tell you what a comfort you've been through all . . . through all this," and her eyes got all watery.

I didn't know what to say, but the prim, punishing voices inside my head that had awakened me that morning, telling me how horribly I'd behaved, were suddenly silent. And, although it would be years before I'd allow myself to act like a human being with patients again, some small part of me heard what this woman was saying, and I would carry this treasure around for years until the time came when I could afford to use it.

But that was years down the line. All I knew at that moment was that my throat was going all tight and achy and I couldn't afford to stay there. So, I mumbled something about having to be somewhere and I got out of there. Fast.

THREE

I GOT through the next couple of months the way an ostrich gets by—by sticking its head in the sand. Only I used surgery instead of sand. I developed a bad case of surgery fever, a disease characterized by a compulsive interest in surgery. It's a disease a lot of residents get, probably for the same reasons that I did.

If I had loved surgery before, now that passion turned into obsession. I breathed freely only in the operating room, and I came to resent the time spent on the ward, in the clinic or on call because it wasn't time spent in OR. I even took to coming into the hospital on my precious few off hours and assisting on operations I hadn't been assigned to.

For some time, I had been drawn to surgery, and now more than ever its concreteness appealed to me. There were so many things inside me that I couldn't touch. Having something outside myself that I could get my hands on fulfilled a need.

Surgery also appealed to me because there was so little human contact, and at that point in my life I wanted things to be impersonal. In truth, however, surgery is not at all impersonal—it is probably the most personal thing one human being can do to another. To probe beneath the skin, to cut open another's belly, to hold the guts in your hands, is to touch someone in the most intensely personal way. But we

44

do our best to make it seem impersonal. We have to, or we wouldn't be able to do it at all.

There are so many taboos in our culture about touching another person's body. If we accidentally brush up against someone in a crowd, we immediately draw back and apologize. Who we may touch, and how, are matters governed by a complex and rigid set of rules. Even the simple act of holding hands is severely restricted, reserved for lovers, young children, and parents with their offspring. To cut open a stranger's body is to violate these taboos in the most extreme way. But we arrange it so that the act is depersonalized in the extreme, thereby allowing ourselves our potentially lethal violations of these taboos.

When we operate, we drape the patient from head to toe in green surgical linens so the only part of the body visible to the surgeon is the operative field. A neurosurgeon, a doctor who operates on the brain, confronts only a bulbous, shaved skull. The rest of the head and the body are hidden from view, which is probably not a bad idea. When you are cutting open a brain and moving into the seat of another person's consciousness, it helps to remain as unconscious as possible of this aspect of what you are doing. When I was an intern working on the neurosurgery ward, the staff doctors experimented briefly with clear plastic surgical drapes. The idea had some merit. It was easier for the anesthesiologist to monitor the patient, to make sure the face didn't grow too pale or the lips turn blue from lack of oxygen. But it was too much for any of us to drill holes in the skull of a person whose face we could see just below the plastic drape, and the see-through drapes were soon abandoned.

In gynecology, we also drape and cover so that all that remains to our view is the one section of the body that we are going to cut into. We abstract the part from the whole. To cut into an abstracted part is possible; to cut into a whole human being is not. But the very capacity for abstraction that makes it possible for us to do our work can also limit us as people. I think it is why so many surgeons are not very good at relating to people.

At any rate, you can see why I was so drawn to surgery at this point in my life. They wheeled the patient in, draped and drugged her, we operated, and they wheeled her out again. We saw her maybe once prior to surgery to do the pre-op medical history and physical, and after surgery for a few moments each morning on rounds until she recovered and went home, and that was that. Things didn't get too sticky or too emotional or too personal. I didn't have any trouble with the Lady of the Lake, and I was thankful for that.

Actually, if I had to have an attack of surgery fever, and apparently I did have to, then I was in the best possible place to have it.

For one thing, there was plenty of surgery to be done. There were hundreds of thousands of members in the prepaid medical plan that I worked for. The members were seen in clinics located throughout the city, as well as in the hospital's own clinics. If someone from an outlying clinic needed surgery, they were referred to the medical plan's central hospital, where I worked. As a result our hospital did a large volume of surgery.

And if I had been at another hospital, there would have been a lot of politics involved in who was going to get to do what surgery there was. At most teaching hospitals, the senior resident in charge of the ward sets up the surgery schedule. He saves the most interesting cases for himself and parcels out to the other residents only those surgeries he's performed often enough to feel entirely confident about. First- or second-year residents working under a senior resident who is greedy or inexperienced may not get to do much more than stand around holding a retractor as third assistant on an operation, which is about as exciting as being a telephone pole. You can't even learn very much that way because, half the time, in order to hold the retractor at the proper angle so the surgeon can see what he is doing, you have to stand in such a way that you can't see what's going on. This wouldn't do much for someone burning up with surgery fever.

There are also lots of politics involved in getting assigned to whatever cases the senior resident decides to pass on to the junior residents. If the senior resident doesn't particularly like you, then you might not get scheduled in OR very often.

Politics of this kind weren't a problem at my hospital, at least not in the OB/GYN department. There were sixteen gynecologists on the staff. Each of the four first-year residents spent a three-month rotation on surgery, as did each of the four third-year residents, and all four second-year residents were assigned to surgery for the entire year. So at any given time there were twenty-two of us handling all the gynecological surgery at the hospital: the sixteen staff doctors, the four second-year residents, and the first- and third-year residents on their three-month surgery rotations. The sixteen staff doctors were divided into groups of four. Every three months, each second-year resident would be assigned to a different one of these four groups, so that by the end of the year, all of us would have spent some time working with each of the staff doctors.

There was a well-defined system for assigning first- and second-year residents to surgery cases. We got assigned to surgical cases in one of two ways. We worked in OB/GYN clinic a couple of afternoons a week and, if we saw a patient in clinic who we thought needed surgery, we referred that patient to one of the four doctors we were assigned to. If that doctor concurred, then the woman was scheduled for surgery and the resident who'd made the initial diagnosis got to assist on the case. Even if one didn't come across clinic patients who needed surgery, there was still ample opportunity to operate, because second-year residents also assisted on the surgeries performed by the four doctors in the group to which he or she was assigned. It was never necessary to play hospital politics or to ingratiate oneself with a senior resident in order to have a chance to get into OR.

Residents burning up with surgery fever are prone to overzealousness. They can be somewhat less than human, and their perspective on things can get dangerously skewed. That patients are people can be overlooked altogether. Patients become bodies to be operated on, opportunities to hone skills. Thank goodness, then, that at the hospital where I worked, the system was set up in such a way that surgery fever couldn't run rampant.

Though the medical profession isn't fond of admitting it, the sad fact remains: There's a lot of unnecessary surgery done in this country, surgery that is done to enrich the surgeon (witness the three hundred thousand unnecessary hysterectomies performed in this country each year). The medical plan where I worked was set up so that there was no advantage to anyone in doing unnecessary surgery. The members of the medical plan paid a flat monthly rate, which covered all their medical expenses. Any operation they might need was covered under that fee. The medical plan itself had nothing to gain from unnecessary surgery. In fact, from the financial point of view, it was better for the plan if there was less, rather than more, surgery. The staff doctors were paid a fixed salary. They got paid the same amount of money regardless of whether they did ten operations a day or one.

There is never a financial incentive for residents to perform unnecessary surgery, because residents, no matter what kind of hospital they are working at, are always paid a fixed salary. Nonetheless, because residents are eager to learn and to develop their surgical skills, they are responsible for a fair share of the unnecessary surgeries that are done. They are not beyond pushing unnecessary surgeries on patients in their zeal to perfect their skills.

It's alarmingly easy to talk women into unnecessary surgery. Say a woman tells a resident that she wants her tubes tied so that she won't get pregnant. Tubal ligation is a relatively minor procedure. The resident may already have done it a hundred times. He knows how to do that procedure, but he may not have done so many hysterectomies. So he tells the woman, "Look, you're finished with your family. You don't need a uterus anymore. Why not have it taken out? It's a simple operation. I can do it through the vagina so you won't even have a visible scar. You'll still look great in a bikini. You won't be bothered by menstrual periods anymore, and you won't ever have to worry about getting uterine cancer."

He may even throw in a few dire statistics about the number of women who get uterine cancer each year. Just the mention of the Big C is enough to scare some women into consenting to surgery. What the resident doesn't tell the woman is that, statistically speaking, she's much more likely to have a complication from the hysterectomy than to develop uterine cancer. He also doesn't tell her that having her uterus removed may affect the intensity of her orgasms.

There are dozens of other ways of talking a woman into having surgery she doesn't need. You can tell her that the fibroid tumor you felt on her uterus during the pelvic exam might be cancer and so, even though she isn't having symptoms, she'd better have it out, "just to be sure." You know that using the word *tumor* is, alone, enough to scare a lot of women into having surgery. What you don't add is that one out of every five women over the age of thirty has a fibroid tumor in her uterus. They're so common that some doctors consider them normal. Nor do you say that, unless they grow so big that they start to cause bothersome tumor symptoms, there's really no need to remove them. In fact, they usually disappear all by themselves after menopause. You also don't inform your patient that the only kind of uterine cancer that could be mistaken for a fibroid is extremely rare and that it would be better just to check her again in a couple of months to see if the tumor has gotten larger (this rare type of cancer grows quickly), than to take her uterus out on the off chance that she has cancer.

There are dozens of similar gambits, but you get the picture.

Often, residents at county hospitals or university affiliated hospitals that cater to the poor are all but running the show. The staff doctors at these hospitals, who usually also have a private practice or appointments to a medical school faculty, generally are not actually at the hospital fulltime. If a resident wants permission to operate, he calls a staff doctor at home and gets the okay by phone. The staff doctor never even sees the patient, so it's fairly easy for the resident to get permission.

You couldn't get away with that sort of thing at our hospital, because all patients had to see a staff doctor for a second opinion before being scheduled for surgery. Also, at our hospital, a staff doctor had to scrub in with the resident. The staff doctors had nothing to gain financially by permitting residents to talk patients into unnecessary surgery; more surgery meant just more work for them.

I like to tell myself that even had I been at another kind of hospital, I wouldn't have done these sorts of things, that I wouldn't have foisted unnecessary surgeries on patients just to satisfy my urge to operate. And, when put like that, I know that of course I would never have done such things; but the forces at work are much subtler than that. Residents who talk patients into unnecessary surgery don't consciously look at them and say to themselves "Aha! I think I'll talk this one into having unnecessary surgery so I'll get a chance to operate"—at least, most of them don't. Like most people, they develop rationalizations for what they're doing.

Suppose a woman has a slightly prolapsed uterus, a fairly common condition (especially among older women who've had a number of children), in which the ligaments that support the uterus are so stretched out that the uterus begins to fall from its normal position. The condition can get so bad that the uterus falls into the vagina or even through the vaginal opening, in which case the uterus has to be removed. But if the uterus is only slightly prolapsed, a woman may live for many years without its becoming a real problem; it may never get so bad that she needs to have her uterus removed. But, the resident tells himself, she'll probably need to have it removed someday, so why not do it now and get it over with? In fact, why not do it *right* now, while I'm here and can do the operation?

If you live and work in an environment where this kind of thinking is acceptable, where it's the norm, then it's easy to fall into that way of looking at things.

It was a good thing that I wasn't in that kind of environment, because once I came down with surgery fever, I'd stay late, volunteering to help on emergency surgeries that came in at night, and in the morning I'd be back in OR, at it again.

The only surgical duty that I didn't embrace wholeheartedly was doing circumcisions. The GYN residents, rather than the pediatrics residents, did the circumcisions on the newborns at our hospital, because we were trained as surgeons and the pediatricians weren't. The four second-year residents took turns, so once every fourth day I was supposed to go over to the newborn nursery and circumcise all the

boy babies that had been born the day before. Sometimes, when the work load in OR got real heavy, the
resident whose turn it was to do circumcisions just
wouldn't get around to it. Then, the resident whose
turn it was the next day would have two days' worth
of babies to circumcise. If no one showed up for a couple of days, they'd start chasing us down. Still, it was
often possible to avoid doing circumcisions, and
whenever I could, I managed to do so. I told myself
that I didn't like doing circumcisions because of the
babies' crying. Besides, it was a simple procedure that
I'd long since mastered. There wasn't anything more
to learn about it. All that was true, but my avoidance
of circumcision also had a lot to do with recalling my
first one. It had been such a horrible experience that
the procedure still had unpleasant associations for
me.

That first circumcision occurred on the very first
day of my internship, which is always a terrible day.
I was scared witless. Working in a hospital as a medical student was one thing, but being an intern was
something else altogether—at least that's how it
seems from a medical student's point of view. Interns
were always dashing about doing terribly important
things; lives hung in the balance. And now I was
going to ascend to this new level of responsibility.
What if I did something wrong? What if someone died
on me? What if I did something so wrong that I killed
someone? Panic, panic. I was Chicken Little and the
sky was falling.

My first day did not get off to an auspicious start. I
reported, bright and early, to the nurses' station in
the middle of the gynecology ward.

"I'm Dr. Patterson, the new intern," I told the
nurse. My voice had the sound of small, brittle things
breaking.

"The new intern?" she said. It was half a question,
half an exclamation of disbelief. She looked at me

doubtfully, suspiciously. "The list says J. Patterson. You . . . you're J. Patterson?"

"That's right. J for Jane, Jane Patterson, Dr. Jane Patterson, see." And I thrust the plastic name tag on my lapel at her.

She was not convinced.

"But, we've never had a woman intern on this floor before." Clearly she did not believe that such an animal existed. I wasn't sure that I did either. I certainly hadn't seen many around. Although they'd had women interns at Prestigious U before me, I was the only woman in my intern class. I mustered up my little breaking-things voice and insisted that I was Dr. Patterson and could she please tell me where to find Dr. Aiken, the first-year resident to whom I was supposed to report. She wasn't very gracious about it, but she did tell me where to find Dr. Aiken.

I found him and, joy of joys, he was a lovely man. "Won't you join us on rounds, Doctor?" he invited. Residents don't as a rule invite interns to do anything. They order them. He said I could call him Gary. I told him to call me Jane. My voice was losing its little breaking-things quality. Maybe the sky wasn't falling after all.

He took me down to the lounge and introduced me to the other intern, Mike Ruffe, who looked as nervous and uncertain as I. But Mike too was very friendly, and said he was glad to know me. We shook hands. It was the last nice thing that happened to me that day.

Gary introduced me to the other residents, who acknowledged me with the merest of grunts. They were busy reviewing the patient charts in preparation for morning rounds.

Morning rounds are a daily ritual in teaching hospitals. All the house staff, the residents and interns, led by a staff doctor, visit the bedside of each patient on the ward. Each patient's case is "presented," that is, someone explains the salient facts about the patient's problems, outlines the diagnostic tests or treatments that have been done so far and their results, describes any complications that may have arisen and suggests plans for further treatment or tests. The job of presenting the case usually falls to the low man, or in this case, the low woman, on the totem pole—the intern—but since this was our first day, the residents presented the cases.

Besides being a way of monitoring patient care, rounds are also a means of teaching medicine. As a medical student, you stuff your head with facts and memorize all that the textbooks have to say about a disease, but real disease in real people doesn't always go by the textbooks. It is on rounds, under the tutelage of an experienced doctor, that you really learn medicine. But the medical hierarchy has a strange way of teaching medicine. There are exceptions, of course, but most of the time, making rounds is a game of one-upmanship. If the intern presents the case succinctly, outlining all the important features of the case and recommending a wise treatment plan, nobody says, "Good, great job." Instead, they start drilling you: What was Mrs. So and So's estrogen level on her last Pap smear? What was her this? What was her that? They keep at you until there's something you don't know, and eventually, there always is. It's a game you can't possibly win, because you're playing against people with vastly more knowledge and experience than you; you're playing against the house. No matter how bright you are or how hard you've studied, there is always some question you can't answer, because you can't know every single detail about every patient. A blood test alone can have some twenty-six different results. You try to remember the three or four serum level results that are relevant to your patient's condition and treatment needs, and you promptly forget the other twenty-three irrelevant ones. Who cares what her serum watermelon level, or whatever, is? It's not relevant.

So, finally, they'll nail you.

"Do you mean you don't know what her serum watermelon level is, Doctor?" they say in a way that implies you've forgotten the most important feature of the case.

"Where did you get your medical training, Doctor?" they ask, and when you tell them, they say, "Aha," in a tone of voice that suggests you might as well have gotten your medical degree from a mail-order correspondence school.

The whole point of all this one-upmanship and constant humiliation is that it's supposed to make you alert, teach you to think on your feet and keep you humble. I suppose the point in making you feel ignorant all the time is to ensure that you don't get so cocky that you get to thinking you know everything and go off doing things on your own when you really should be asking for help. And, part of this questioning is legitimate. Your superiors have to know how good you are and exactly what you know and don't know before they can trust you with an increased level of responsibility. But there must be better ways to achieve the same effects. As it is, energy is wasted and things get very confusing, because usually it's hard to tell whether they're just playing get-the-intern or whether the question you just said "I don't know" to truly is something you need to know in order to take care of that patient.

The doctor I made rounds with that first day was from the set-'em-up-and-knock-'em-down school of medical education. I'd seen it happen to others, but I had never before been on the receiving end. When he started in on me that day, I felt my knees go all shaky and my voice get all little and unsteady again. No intern could be expected to know the answers to the questions that he was firing at me, but I didn't know

that then. My continuous string of I-don't-know-sirs
made me feel like an idiot, an undereducated one.

By the time we'd finished rounds, I wanted to run
crying home to mommy, but mommy was three thousand miles away and I had to go up to surgery to assist on an operation. All I did in surgery was hold a
retractor the whole time. The surgeon kept yelling at
me to hold the retractor properly, but I didn't know
what I was doing wrong. If I'd been a little less intimidated, I would have realized that I wasn't doing anything wrong. If I had really been doing something
wrong, he would have had to tell me how to do it
right or he wouldn't have been able to go on with
the surgery. He had just run into some trouble with
the operation and was blowing off some steam on the
nearest convenient peon, the intern—standard operating procedure. But, I didn't know that either, and I
left the operating room feeling like a complete failure.

Then I had to go back down to the ward and do all
the tasks I'd been assigned during rounds. I had
twenty-some patients assigned to me. Each one
needed some sort of test or procedure, and I didn't
even know where to start. I had one woman who had
been operated on three days before who hadn't uri-
nated on her own since the operation. I was supposed
to catheterize her, put a tube up her urethra into her
bladder and drain the urine from her bladder. That
seemed high priority, so I decided to do that first.

One of the cardinal rules for patients is: Never get
sick during the first week of July. July is the beginning
of the medical year. Internships start on July first; res-
idencies start on July first; staff doctors' contracts run
from July first to July first. Chances are that most, if
not all, of the doctors on the floor are new to the
ward. No one knows where anything is except the
nurses, the aides and the orderlies. You are completely at their mercy as they are the only ones who
know where the instruments are kept or where the

forms for the blood laboratory requisitions are or how
to send a specimen down to the lab for urinalysis. As
a result, everyone is running around like electrified
chickens, and chaos reigns.

One of the nurses' aides told me where to find the
sterile gloves I needed for the catheterization, but she
didn't know where the catheters were kept. The
nurse knew, but she took her time telling me. Then I
managed to get an orderly to show me where to find
the adhesive tape I needed to tape the urine collection
bag to the woman's leg. When I finally got all the stuff
together and went into her room to do the procedure,
the lady with the full bladder kept insisting that I
wasn't her doctor, that Dr. Taylor, that "nice young
man" was. I explained that I was the new intern, and
I was taking Dr. Taylor's place. She clearly didn't approve of the substitution.

The urine collection bag was a little different from
the ones I'd used in medical school, and I wasn't
quite sure how to attach it to the catheter tube. I fumbled with it until I thought I had it right. The woman
was glaring at me the whole time. As I inserted the
catheter, she moaned and complained, probably with
good cause, as I was hardly an expert.

The urine hit the collection bag full force, detaching
the bag from the tube. (I hadn't hooked it up properly.) The urine poured out on the floor as I hopped
about, trying to keep my feet out of it while apolo-
gizing to the woman.

Finally, I found an orderly, and he mopped it up,
looking down his nose at me the whole time. Somehow I managed to bumble my way through the next
several hours. Even the ward clerk got a chance to hit
on me that day. I didn't know how to work the credit
card-type machine that was used to stamp the lab
requisition slips, so she had to teach me. It took me
until six o'clock to finish my work. I hadn't eaten
lunch or dinner, because there hadn't been any time.

Besides, I didn't know where the cafeteria was. I was tired and hungry and about to go home when I heard my name being paged.

I picked up the page phone. It was a nurse from the newborn nursery.

"You have five circumcisions to do," she said.

"Circumcisions?" This was the last straw in a day that would have broken any camel's back. "What are you talking about? I'm the GYN intern. I've never even seen a circumcision, let alone done one." I was fairly screaming into the receiver.

"Well, Dr. Patterson . . . this is *Dr.* Patterson, isn't it?"

"Yes," I acknowledged reluctantly.

"Well, you have five circumcisions to do." And she hung up on me.

Frantically, I paged the other intern, Mike Ruffe.

"What'll I do? They want me to come over to the newborn nursery and do five circumcisions. I've never even seen a circumcision."

"No problem," said Mike. "Meet me in the nursery in ten minutes, and I'll show you how. Nothing to it."

We scrubbed and put on sterile gowns and gloves. I watched, wide-eyed, as Mike did a circumcision on the first baby.

"Okay, Jane, you've seen one, now do one," Mike said.

This is known as the see-one, do-one, teach-one philosophy of medicine. It's supposed to be a joke, an exaggeration. Ideally, you should see a procedure several times, assist in doing it a number of times, and then, finally, with supervision, do the procedure yourself. Eventually, after you've done it many, many times, you should be able to teach someone else to do it. But it doesn't always happen the ideal way, in the catch-as-catch-can world of ward medicine.

The nurse brought this little baby in and put him

into a cutout contraption known as a Circumstraint, spreading his arms and legs wide apart and fastening his limbs down with the restraining straps. He looked for all the world like a sacrificial offering or a crucifixion candidate. I washed the penis and scrotum with antiseptic solution and placed a round surgical drape over his groin.

The first step in doing a circumcision is freeing up the foreskin. This is done by inserting a blunt probe beneath the foreskin and moving it around so that any little adhesions that might cause the foreskin to adhere to the penis will be broken up. This may sound simple enough, but you can do all sorts of things wrong, like inserting the probe into the urethra instead of under the foreskin. Ouch. I managed not to do this.

Next, you take a clamp and insert the blade of the clamp under the foreskin. Then, you bring the blades of the clamp together, catching a vertical strip of foreskin between the blades. Squeeze. Hard.

We perform this barbaric procedure because studies have shown that uncircumcised men have a higher incidence of cancer of the penis than circumcised men.

The theory is that the nervous system of the newborn is not yet fully developed and, therefore, the baby doesn't feel much pain. Interesting theory, but you couldn't prove it by me. In my experience, they all scream bloody murder.

Next you remove the clamp. The skin that has been caught between the blades of the clamp is smashed flat, tissue-paper thin. Then you take a pair of scissors and cut a straight line down the center of the tissue-thin skin that has been flattened by the pressure of the blades. Now, if he's not already at it, the baby sets up a caterwaul. There's very little bleeding, because the pressure of the clamp has closed off the blood vessels in the area. Then you fold the foreskin back down over itself as though you were peeling a miniature banana.

Next you place a tiny, hollow, bell-shaped instrument over the exposed glans of the penis. Then you bring the split foreskin back up over the bell, as if you were putting the peel back on the banana.

Now comes the tough part. A second instrument is placed over the foreskin and the bell. The second instrument has a small hole in the top through which you must tug at the foreskin, pulling it up so that it is taut and even all around and won't slip back down. Then you tighten down the screw clamp on the second instrument. Another yelp from baby. The foreskin, caught between the two instruments, is smashed flat, and the blood vessels in the area are thereby squeezed closed. Then you draw your scalpel all along the top edge of the bell, cutting away the foreskin. Remove the two instruments and, presto, you've done a circumcision. Easy as pie. It takes only five minutes.

Forty-five minutes later, I had completed my first circumcision. The baby was howling. I was drenched with sweat.

"Not bad," Mike yelled encouragingly, over the baby's howling.

"Try telling him that," I yelled back.

The next one was a little better. It only took a half hour. I whizzed through baby number four in fifteen minutes. I was practically an expert.

"Nice going. You're a regular Zorro with that blade." Mike was trying to cheer me up. "Hey, know what? You're the first person I ever taught to do a circumcision," he told me proudly.

This soon became evident. Mike had forgotten to tell me I should check under the instrument after it's tightened down, as it's possible to catch something other than the foreskin up inside the bell. I slashed away with my blade on baby number five, removed the bell, and there was blood everywhere. For a terrible, adrenaline-surging moment, I thought, "I've castrated him!"

I hadn't. What I'd done was to cut the media raphe, the ridge of skin at the juncture of the scrotal sacs, which I'd inadvertently caught up in the bell. It was just a little nick, but bloody. A couple of quick zigzag stitches and baby was back together again, which was more than I could say for myself.

"Jesus, Mike, what are we going to tell the mother?" I said.

"No problem," said Mike, "we'll tell her it's the Mark of Zorro."

That had been my first day on circumcision and my first and last Mark of Zorro. Still, the Mark of Zorro was always in the back of my mind whenever I did a circumcision, and I avoided them whenever possible.

One day in early March, just about the time that I first came down with surgery fever, I was paged over to the newborn nursery to do circumcisions. No one had been there in a couple of days, and there were a lot of babies to be circumcised, which didn't make me very happy; but I had to do it. While I was working, Dr. Wright, one of the four surgeons I was assigned to at the time, happened to come into the nursery.

"No, no, no," he cried when he saw what I was doing. "That's terrible, just terrible. You don't do this well at all. You must never, never spill a drop of blood during a circumcision, not a single drop!"

I was rather put out by his criticism. I considered myself fairly adept at the procedure. Besides, I didn't agree with him. It *is* possible to do a circumcision without spilling a single drop of blood, but it takes three times as long. If you want to avoid any blood loss whatsoever, you have to increase the pressure on the clamp and tighten the instrument as much as possible, and you have to keep the pressure on longer so that all the blood vessels in the area are totally flattened out. But why prolong the baby's agony? A healthy infant isn't going to miss a drop of blood.

I didn't, of course, argue the point with Dr. Wright. He was the teacher, I was the student. The medical hierarchy is a lot like a military bureaucracy. There are the generals, who are the surgeons, and there are the privates, the residents. Generals give orders and privates follow them. Just as privates do not argue the merits of their orders, residents do not argue with surgeons.

Dr. Wright made me do the rest of the circumcisions his way. The whole time, he was breathing down my neck and lecturing me about not spilling a drop of blood. We didn't spill a drop of blood, but the whole nursery was ringing with the cries of the screaming infants. After that, I religiously avoided Dr. Wright.

Actually, I had already been avoiding him whenever possible. Like the other residents, I always referred my clinic patients who needed surgery to one of the other three surgeons I was assigned to, because Dr. Wright was peculiar, even to the point of being bizarre. He had a reputation for being meticulous, and it was well deserved. He was more than meticulous, he was downright maniacal, and about the strangest things. One time, when I'd gotten stuck operating with him, he went berserk about the way I'd put the surgical drapes on the patient. He made me take the drapes off, and spent a half hour showing me the absolutely proper and precise way to drape a patient. I couldn't believe he was being so fussy about it. Not only was precision draping unimportant; he was doing all this adjusting while the patient was under anesthesia. The longer a patient stays under anesthesia, the greater the risks of developing a complication. You don't want to hurry during surgery, but you certainly don't waste time on surgical drapes.

Even though I tried, it wasn't always possible to

avoid referring clinic patients to Dr. Wright and thus having to operate with him, because there were inevitably occasions when the schedules of the other three surgeons I was assigned to were filled. Also, if Dr. Wright saw patients in clinic who needed surgery or had cases referred in from the outlying clinics, he could request assistance in surgery, and if your OR schedule wasn't full, you might get stuck operating with him.

Dr. Wright was as meticulous about the actual surgery as he was about details like the drapes. He wasn't a bad surgeon as far as technique was concerned, but he was slow. He was a fanatic about blood loss. He'd open up an abdomen to do a hysterectomy, and then he'd spend an extra half hour or hour or even more tying off all the blood vessels. He'd tie off a vessel, and then he'd stop and wait for a few minutes and check and recheck every blood vessel to make sure there wasn't any leakage. Now, it's all very well and good to be concerned about blood loss during surgery, but he took it too far. There's a trade-off here. If you wait five minutes every time you tie off a vessel to make sure it won't leak, the patient isn't going to lose as much blood during the operation as she would otherwise, but you've significantly extended the operating time and thus the time under anesthesia, which is a lot riskier.

Once my surgery fever hit full stride, I actually volunteered to stay at the hospital on one of my afternoons off. Dr. Wright had an operation scheduled that day, and his assistant was tied up in another surgery, so I agreed to help out. The operation was an ovarian cystectomy, an operation to remove a cyst from the ovary. The length of time it takes to do a cystectomy varies depending on the size of the cyst and a number of other factors, but assuming it's just a simple cyst, the operation normally takes about forty-five minutes. The cystectomy we did that day was a rou-

tine case, but it took two and a half hours. Every time
we tied off a blood vessel, Dr. Wright would stop and
watch the vessel for a few minutes to make sure there
wasn't going to be any blood seepage. And he kept
making me put in extra stitches here and there because he imagined that he'd seen a little blood somewhere. It was possibly the most tedious piece of
surgery I'd ever done.

What I should have done at that point was go to
the chief and inform him about Dr. Wright's methods. But so far, I'd only seen him operate on young,
healthy patients who could withstand such treatment, and, I told myself, he might have different
standards when operating on someone at high risk
for anesthesia complications.

And so I did nothing. I was too much under the
sway of the medical hierarchy. I told myself that he
was the teacher and I was just the student. Who was I
to criticize? Which is no excuse. In particular, it was
no excuse for me, because I had been through a similar experience the previous July, at the very beginning
of the second year of my residency, and the chief had
been very clear with me about where my responsibility lay. The previous situation had been with a surgeon named Dr. Collins. I was doing my first vaginal
hysterectomy. I had assisted on vaginal hysterectomies before, but for the first time I was actually the
surgeon in charge of the case. I had just started the
operation and was seated between the woman's legs,
beginning the incision. Dr. Collins, acting as first assistant, was standing to my right, and one of the first-
year residents, second assistant, was standing to my
left. Making the incision in the vagina to get into the
pelvic cavity so that you can get at the uterus is a little
tricky, and I was having some trouble with it. Instead
of giving me some advice or moving into my seat and
taking over the operation, Dr. Collins grabbed the
scalpel out of my hand and began cutting, his hands

all shaky. He was still standing at my side, and from that position it's impossible to see what you're doing, but he kept slashing away. He had the knife in one hand and the suction in the other, but he was too busy cutting to do any suctioning. The woman was bleeding profusely, and he couldn't possibly have seen what he was doing for all the blood.

At that point we had to transfuse the woman with two units of blood. Normally, transfusion is unnecessary in a vaginal hysterectomy—and this was just the beginning of the operation and we'd already had to give her two units. I don't know what would have happened to that woman if it hadn't been for the nurse. She saw what was going on and paged for another staff doctor, who came in and took my place. I took over Dr. Collins's place as first assistant, and together we finished up the operation while Dr. Collins went out into the lounge and smoked a cigarette.

I knew I should have gone to the chief and said something about Dr. Collins. I couldn't count on the staff doctor talking to the chief, because he had come in in the middle of the thing and didn't really know what had happened. But I didn't go to the chief, partly because I felt what had happened was somehow my fault. And I thought, well, maybe Dr. Collins was just having a bad day, and it didn't seem that anyone should be called down for having one bad day. Still, I made sure I never scrubbed with him again. And soon I began to hear through the grapevine that these kinds of incidents were happening with other residents when they worked with Dr. Collins. Apparently someone else finally went to the chief and said something, because one afternoon he called me into his office and asked me about Dr. Collins.

"I'm glad you asked me about him," I said, "because I never want to scrub with him again," and I told the chief what had happened. He was furious.

"Why didn't you come to me immediately as soon as that happened?" he yelled.

"No excuse, sir," was all I could say.

Dr. Collins's surgical privileges were suspended, and supposedly I had learned something about my responsibility in such situations.

Apparently I hadn't, because, despite the experience with Dr. Collins, I did not go to the chief about Dr. Wright. I had spent too many years knuckling under in an authoritarian system to have the stuff to defy that system, even though it should have been clear to me that the chief would have listened. Instead, I told myself that the Wright and Collins situations were different from one another. As far as I knew, Dr. Wright hadn't endangered anyone's life. Besides, no one else was saying anything, so maybe I was wrong about him.

At first only the residents were in a position to know what was going on, because we were the only ones who operated with him. But then things got worse. Dr. Wright got slower. He'd be scheduled for a forty-five-minute operation at seven o'clock, and three hours later he'd still be in OR. He was throwing off the whole OR schedule and delaying other surgeons' cases. They'd get mad and yell at him.

"Well, there were a lot of bleeders on that case, and it took a long time to get all those little bleeders tied off," he'd explain, and he got away with it. I guess it didn't happen that he delayed any one surgeon's operations enough times to tip anyone off to what was really going on.

But then things got still worse. Dr. Wright began calling for a second staff doctor to look at his work before he'd close an incision. "Is this okay?" he'd want to know. "Does everything look all right here?"

The staff doctor would look and say, "Sure, sure. Everything looks fine. Why don't you close? What's the problem?"—and sort of shrug his shoulders and walk away, no doubt wondering what was troubling the guy. But no one did anything about it, or even recognized that Dr. Wright had a serious problem. He slipped through the net because he was a general, because when you get to the top of the medical bureaucracy, you're beyond scrutiny.

And then, one Thursday afternoon while we were all at educational conference, Dr. Wright went home and then out to his garage. He put a plastic bag over his head, meticulously tying it around his neck with a series of precise surgical knots. Then he put a gun up inside the plastic bag and shot himself.

Even to the end he was meticulous, using the plastic bag, because you don't spill a drop of blood when you do a circumcision and you don't spill a drop of blood when you kill yourself either.

FOUR

A COUPLE of weeks after Dr. Wright's suicide, I ran into one of the surgery residents on the medicine ward. Actually, he ran into me. He was charging down the hall, and he almost knocked me over.

"Look, look what I've got," he demanded gleefully, waving a fistful of papers in my face.

I looked. He had a bunch of the pink triplicate forms that we used when we transferred a patient from one ward to another.

"I got five thyroids from Medicine. *Five* of them, and they're all mine!" He was fairly writhing with excitement.

He meant that five patients with thyroid problems who had been getting drug therapy on the medicine ward were going to be transferred to the surgery ward. Presumably, the medical approach to treating their thyroid conditions hadn't been successful, so now they were going to have to undergo surgery. Somehow he'd managed to get all five patients, so he'd get to assist on their surgeries. Five thyroid surgeries—riches beyond a resident's wildest dreams, and he'd managed to snag them all.

I stood there looking into the face of his ghoulish enthusiasm, which was devoid of compassion for the five people who were going to have to undergo this terrible, debilitating surgery, and it was comic in a black humor sort of way. All I could think of was *Dr. Strangelove*, the movie in which a crazed general pushes the red button and launches a nuclear attack on the Russkies. There's no way to call back the plane with the bomb, and the Russians' nuclear defense system is completely automated, so they have no way of stopping their bombs from retaliating, and the whole world is going to blow up. At the end of the movie, all the generals and the ambassadors and the President are in the war room at the Pentagon, and Peter Sellers is playing the demented Germanic science advisor. They've all just realized that the world is about to be annihilated, and are sitting there looking at each other. The Sellers character, Dr. Strangelove, starts to speak, telling them that it's all okay because there's a contingency plan, a secret underground headquarters, fully stocked for Doomsday, complete with luscious blond nymphets, three young blondes for every man, and this is an opportunity to breed a new Aryan race from the ashes of human civilization. While he explains this, more and more of his true, crazed nature shows through: As he talks, his crippled left arm keeps spasming up into a fascist salute. He tries to hold it down with his right hand. Finally he can no longer control it, and he finishes his master-race speech doing a full-on Nazi salute, to which all respond by rising to their feet and saluting back, drooling over the idea of luscious blondes and endless sex, having lost sight of the fact that the world is about to end. It's a hideously funny scene, and it sprang wide-screen into my head as I stood looking at this resident.

"Hey, well, yeah, that's terrific," I said. "What a piece of luck. Five thyroid surgeries is good news. It's better than a ten-victim freeway pileup rolling into ER." But my sarcasm went right by him.

"Oh, much better," he agreed. "The senior residents hog all the good ones in car accidents. I'm lucky if I get a serious surface wound."

He went off down the hall, and I went home and looked at myself in the mirror. Did I have that same mad gleam in my eye?

The terrible thing about the whole encounter was that I understood all too well where he was coming from—and the neighborhood was mine. I wasn't quite as far gone as he was, but I was intimately acquainted with that surge of inhuman glee you get when you've been fortunate enough to find a ''good'' gynecological surgery case.

I did not like what I was seeing in my mirror.

I started thinking about Dr. Wright's suicide. I had been telling myself that Wright was mad. He was an obsessive/compulsive neurotic who'd slipped over that fine line into a psychotic episode, and whammo. That was really all there was to it. I was shocked by his suicide, and, of course, saddened. Here had been a human being, obviously in great distress, and no one around him had helped him or had even recognized that he was in need of help. But that was as far as I went with my thoughts at the time. Dr. Wright's suicide didn't seem to have anything to do with me or what was going on in my life.

Now, pondering my fellow resident's fiendish enthusiasm about the thyroid operations and seeing in myself much the same unhealthy absorption in surgery, I felt for a moment that Dr. Wright's suicide was not just the isolated, unconnected act of one crazy individual, but the madly logical consequence of our surgical training. I had a sudden vision of surgeons as people so insanely intent on pursuing scientific knowledge that they lose all humanity, like a gang of Dr. Frankensteins.

It wasn't a pleasant thought, so I shook it off, dismissing it as another of my paranoid flashes. I am always exaggerating, I reminded myself, always making too much of things. Still, after that, my surgery fever cooled off; at least I stopped coming by the hospital on my off hours.

Now that I wasn't hanging around the hospital so much, there was a problem about what to do with my free hours. It wasn't a huge problem, because there weren't very many off hours to fill. I was on duty from seven o'clock every morning until my work was finished. I was frequently at the hospital until seven at night, and at times even later. Rarely would I get off at four or five. Every fourth night I was on call, which meant I had to stay at the hospital until seven o'clock the next morning, at which time I'd start my regular day shift. We also worked half days on Saturdays. On Monday evenings, a residents' conference kept us at the hospital until nine o'clock at night. I was also on duty every fourth Sunday. We had one afternoon a week off, plus one half day Saturday and three Sundays a month. Beyond that, we were also expected to read all the medical journals and keep up on all the latest developments in the field. One evening each month was taken up by a meeting at the chief's house, where we'd present summaries of the journal articles we'd read in the preceding weeks.

It was a demanding schedule. Throw in things like brushing your teeth and taking out the trash, and that pretty much filled up your life. Still, there was a little time left for socializing.

But I didn't have anybody to socialize with. I had moved clear across the country, and I knew only the people I worked with. Most of the other residents were married or had girlfriends. They got together socially from time to time, but always as couples, doing couple things. The other residents were all guys, and once in a while they'd have a sort of boys' night out, and one or two of the staff doctors would join them. They invited me along a couple of times, but I wasn't one of the boys. They'd have a few beers and start talking about this patient who had a "really great set of knockers" or that one who "came on" to them while they were doing a pelvic exam. That brand of shop talk embarrassed me and, once they'd realized what they'd said in front of me, embarrassed them too. I took to politely declining their invitations, which made us all feel more comfortable.

So I'd sit at home alone reading my medical journals. I was lonely, but I'd been lonely for a long time, ever since I'd started medical school. It hadn't been quite so bad in medical school, because I had gone to college in the same town where I went to medical school, so I'd still see some of my college friends now and then. But our interests had diverged. They were all engaged and about to get married, or were married and having kids.

There were a few other women in my class at medical school, but I never got to know any of them well. Three of them had dropped out by the end of the second year. That left only two other women besides me, out of a class of one hundred and seven, who made it all the way through. I lived at home and they lived on campus, so there was no living together, none of that late-night-studying camaraderie in the dorms to draw us together. Besides, I didn't particularly like them. I didn't dislike them, but I didn't feel drawn to them either, so we never grew close.

Still, I wasn't entirely alone in my medical school days. In fact I was engaged for the first two years. My fiancé, a bacteriologist, lived in upstate New York, a good two hundred miles from my medical school; but we'd fly back and forth on weekends sometimes, and we'd see each other on holidays. I broke the engagement at the beginning of my third year of medical school, and I suppose it must have been a gut-wrenchingly miserable time for me, but when I look back on it now, all I can remember are the humorous aspects.

My fiancé liked things to go his way, and he became

vindictive when they didn't, which had a lot to do with why I ended the engagement. Then he was so mad at me for breaking the engagement—not so much out of love for me as out of rage that I had thwarted his plans—that he sued me for "return of gifts given in expectation of matrimony." There was some archaic law still on the books that derived from the days when women brought dowries to their marriages. When the dowry involved, as it often did, a herd of cows, a piece of land, ten good laying hens and a mule, the intended husband would often take possession of the goodies and start managing the livestock and the land prior to the marriage. If a lovers' spat or some other problem canceled the marriage plans, the woman's father could, under this law, sue to get the dowry back so he'd have some assets with which to stake another attempt at matrimony for his daughter.

My fiancé had given me a microscope, a wonderful high-tech instrument, one I couldn't have afforded myself. I had to have a microscope for medical school, and without his gift I would have been stuck with a bruised and abused microscope discarded from a high school biology lab. Still I think I would have just given it back, if it hadn't been for the lawsuit. He not only sued me for the return of the microscope, he wanted it returned in the same condition in which he'd given it to me. That is, he wanted me to buy him a new microscope. He also wanted about ten other things, including reimbursement for the plane tickets he'd paid for when I'd visited him in New York.

You can't get blood from a stone, and I didn't have any money. Luckily, the case never got to court. My attorney told me that, not only was this the first time a suit evoking this law had been put before the courts since 1902, but it was also the only time a man had ever brought suit against a woman under this law. A real feminist first.

At any rate, at the height of our legal entangle-
ments, my by then ex-fiancé took to showing up at
the medical school and creating loud scenes in front of
everyone. If I'd thought his dramatics had anything
to do with affection for me, I might at least have given
the microscope back. But as it was, I held on to it, provoked further scenes, and so developed a rather scar-
let reputation; I was a woman who drove men to
dangerous extremes. I was not exactly plagued by requests for dates during the remainder of my medical
school career.

The loneliness got a lot more intense once I began
my internship. I had moved out to the West Coast;
the only people I knew were other interns; the demands of internship left little time for socializing; I
was the only woman in the class. I was alone.

After my internship, I was the only woman resident
at the hospital, and although I had by then resigned
myself to the loneliness and alienation, I still felt at
times like a freak. I suppose I should have realized all
along that a woman going into medicine was bound
to feel lonely, that I would always be one of only a few
women in a man's world, but during childhood I had
picked up the notion that there was nothing at all unusual or out of the way about being a woman doctor.
Like most notions picked up in childhood, this one
had a remarkable tenacity, and it wasn't until fairly
late in the game that it came home to me that there
weren't a lot of women doctors around.

It was probably just as well that it took me till late in
the game to realize that being a woman doctor was a
pioneering ambition, because I am not by tempera-
ment a pioneer. Let other, more courageous types
blaze new trails. I prefer to follow along behind at a
comfortable distance and on well-trodden paths.

The reason it took me so long to catch on to the fact
that there weren't exactly hordes of women doctors
around was Fred. Fred was my brother, nine years

my senior, and always the person in our family to whom I was closest. It was he to whom I turned when I needed help or emotional support. He counseled and consoled me and dried up all my tears. I, in turn, accorded him the status of a minor god and fell into the habit of considering everything he said as gospel truth.

One day, I must have been ten or eleven, Fred sat me down and asked me what I wanted to be when I grew up. Growing up was light-years away as far as I was concerned, and I wasn't even sure I was planning on doing it.

"Uh, I dunno," I answered with preadolescent élan. But I'd been around long enough to know which way the wind was blowing. I knew the options for females in the fifties.

"A nurse or a teacher?" I guessed.

My brother, God bless him, had a counteroffer. "Well, why not a doctor or a professor? You know, Janey, just because you're a girl doesn't mean anything. Girls can be anything they want to be."

We talked it over, and I decided if that was the case, I guessed I'd like to be a doctor. (I was good in science, and besides, Fred had just started medical school.) And that was that. From then on, any time kindly adults leaned over, patted me on the head and asked me what I wanted to be when I grew up, I told them I was going to be a doctor.

From time to time, well-meaning relatives or school-teachers would try to discourage me. Their intentions were honorable. They sincerely believed that, as a woman, I would be happier aspiring to be a mother and a housewife, or, if I was hell-bent on a career, a librarian, a teacher, or the like. I didn't pay much attention to these efforts to sidetrack me into an occupation considered better suited to my gender. I figured Fred just hadn't gotten around to telling them how girls could be anything they wanted to be.

By the time I got to college, I was announcing my career plans with such conviction that no one bothered trying to discourage me anymore. Even though I couldn't have failed to notice by then that there weren't very many women doctors around, somehow this fact didn't register. I went to a women's college. The emphasis in women's colleges then was still on educating women for "gracious living" so that we'd become pillars of the community and good wives to the doctors and lawyers we were supposed to marry. Still, the idea of a woman pursuing a career for herself wasn't totally alien to that environment, and I guess I applied to medical school expecting that a fair number of other women out there were doing the same thing.

I applied to three schools in the fall of my senior year without having yet grasped the fact that I was entering a man's world. I think it first began to hit me during my medical school interviews, which did not go at all well. At one school I was interviewed by a panel of doctors. As I remember it, there were dozens of doctors in this huge room who fired questions at me for hours. Actually, there probably were no more than three or four doctors in, at best, a medium-sized office, and the interview couldn't have lasted more than forty-five minutes.

Most of their questions ran along the lines of, "Did I have a boyfriend?" "Was I engaged?" "Did I plan to get married and have children?" They didn't, of course, ask such questions of male applicants. Incidentally, they don't (or aren't supposed to) ask them of women anymore either, because it's now illegal to do so. But it would be almost another decade before there was serious talk about an Equal Rights Amendment, before there would be any Affirmative Action Programs, before anyone would even begin to make nervous jokes about "women's libbers." It would never have occurred to me to challenge my interviewers' right to ask these questions. All I was concerned

about was getting the right answers, which I was beginning to realize might be rather tricky. I wanted to
sound like a normal, feminine female, but I also
wanted to let them know that I was serious about a career and that my career came first. That was not easy
to do in those days. Being feminine and career-
oriented was a contradiction in terms.

The significance of the drift of their questions did
not entirely escape me. When springtime rolled
around and I still hadn't heard from any of the
schools, it began to dawn on me that, not only might
there not be very many other women in my class at
medical school, but I might not be there either. And
then what would I do? I didn't have any second
choices. All I had ever wanted to do was be a doctor.
Just as real panic was about to set in, I received accep-
tance notices from all three schools. In the end, I
chose a university near my hometown in order to live
with my parents and save myself a lot of financial
problems.

Being one of the few women in a man's world, I'd
found it a long and lonely haul, but I'd pretty much
resigned myself to it. Then, one day during the spring
of my second year of residency, one of the nurses casually mentioned that she and a bunch of the other
nurses got together on Friday nights for a few drinks,
and why didn't I come along? Any social graces I
might ever have possessed had long since fallen into
such disuse that I could only splutter in stunned surprise at the unexpected invitation, making her think I
was reluctant to accept.

"Oh, come on," she urged. "We have a good ole
time. A regular hen's party—just us girls—you know,
a girls' night out."

Going out with the girls became a regular Friday
night ritual with me, and we did have a good ole time.
We'd have a few beers and talk about the things
women always talk about—lovers, kids, our prob-

lems, our jobs, what we were mad about, what we were glad about, how we felt about things. Woman talk was almost an alien language to me. I had been talking medicalese for so long—that objective, bloodless, scientific man talk—that I was tongue-tied at first. I had no language for talking about interior landscapes.

Now that I look back on it, I can see that what I was doing in those beer bars with a gaggle of women on Friday nights was learning how to talk to myself again; but all I knew then was that I was talking woman talk, and that it felt good.

When I discussed a case with my male colleagues, we talked about the fibroid tumor in Room 403 or the inoperable uterine cancer in Room 507. But on girls' night out, the fibroid tumor in Room 403 was Mrs. Johnson, and wasn't it sad that she was going to lose her uterus and wouldn't be able to have any kids and she was only twenty-seven? And the uterine cancer in Room 507 was Mrs. Jones, and wasn't it terrible that this dear old woman was dying and none of her no-good kids ever came in to visit her?

Not that these nurses were always such angels of mercy. They'd bitch on and on about a "demanding old bat" who was always turning on her light so the nurse would come in the room and hold the Kleenex while she blew her nose, or about some young snip who'd want them to come in and remake her bed because the corners weren't tucked in neatly enough. And they'd complain endlessly about the endless complaints they heard: "My back hurts." "My breakfast was cold." "The doctor didn't talk to me enough." "My ice water's lukewarm." "My pillow's uncomfortable." "This isn't right." "That's wrong." . . . Whine, kvetch, complain. But, whether they were being sympathetic or grousing about a patient, they always talked about patients as human beings, not conditions.

After a couple of beers, the conversation would inevitably come around to their main gripe: the doctors.

"You know what Dr. Phillips did to me today? The meal trays came up from the cafeteria late. I was running around like a madwoman trying to get everyone their lunch, and I hear Phillips yelling, 'Nurse, nurse, I need a nurse in here!' So, I race in there, and he says, 'Cut me a piece of tape.' He's standing there with the scissors and the tape right in his hand. But, instead of cutting it himself, he hands it to me to cut. I wanted to cut *him*."

"Oh, I know, Susan," Ginny would say. "Dr. Jacks pulled the same number on me—'Nurse, nurse, I want a nurse!'—and you know what he wanted? He wanted me to remove a Band-Aid for him. A surgeon, with two perfectly good hands, and he calls me in to remove a Band-Aid."

I could understand their complaints, because I was often mistaken for a nurse. I'd be sitting at the nurses' station writing orders, and a staff doctor or a resident would come along and tell me to get up because he wanted to sit down. Then he'd see my stethoscope and realize my white uniform was a doctor's coat, not a nurse's uniform, and he'd apologize, "Oh, I'm sorry. I thought you were a nurse," as if that were adequate explanation for his rudeness.

"That's not news to me," grumped Susan. "I'm only surprised he didn't ask you to shine his shoes while he was sitting there."

I'd been on the receiving end of such treatment often enough that I knew how it felt, and I tried not to behave that way myself. If I was in the room seeing a patient, and she needed a bedpan, I'd get it for her. It was easier as well as quicker just to do it myself, but a lot of doctors would call in a nurse. Maybe the male doctors felt a female patient would be embarrassed if he put her on a bedpan. But they'd stand right there and watch while the nurse did it. I think it was mostly that they thought bedpans beneath their dignity.

The first couple of times we got together and the nurses started complaining about doctors, I felt myself shrinking back in my seat: These women were really mad, and they were mad at doctors, and I was a doctor. But, then, one evening as they were warming up for a round of ''You know what Dr. So and So did to me,'' one of the nurses turned to me and said, ''That's why it's so nice having a woman doctor around. You don't do that kind of shit.''

''Well, Jane doesn't,'' said another one, ''but that's just 'cause of who she is. There was a woman doctor on the staff where I trained, and she was ten times worse than any male doctor.'' The conversation veered off into a can-you-top-this comparison of who was generally more horrible—men or women doctors. But at least it was firmly established that in this them-against-us battle, I wasn't a them, which made me feel good.

During this time, when I was beginning to hang out with the nurses, something happened to me that would have a profound influence on me as a doctor. I woke up one morning after a night out with the girls feeling as if my vagina had suddenly turned to lead. I also had sharp pains in my lower abdomen. I immediately panicked: I had some rare and virulent form of gynecological cancer and would be dead by nightfall. But after reviewing my own case, and the dearth of other symptoms, I realized that I was having my very first attack of menstrual cramps.

I put my hands on my belly and stared at myself in wonderment, the way some women do when you inform them they're pregnant. So there really was such a thing after all! I had never quite believed in them before, largely because I had never felt them before. I'd started to menstruate at a normal age and had been chugging along like clockwork every month since then with nary a twinge of pain. When I was a kid in junior high and high school, I would hear other girls complaining about their cramps, but I never took them seriously. For one thing, they seemed to enjoy complaining about it so much. Besides, if you complained enough, you could sometimes work it up into an excuse for getting out of gym class. Of course that always infuriated the gym teacher, who considered menstrual cramps a form of female malingering. I was on the gym teacher's side.

My medical school education reinforced the it's-all-in-your-head theory of menstrual cramps. Medical science isn't much more sophisticated about cramps than my gym teacher was. Oh, medicine has a fancier name for it. They call it dysmenorrhea, of which there are two kinds.

Secondary dysmenorrhea is menstrual pain associated with some underlying disease. A woman might, for instance, have a fibroid tumor in her uterus. If the tumor is located in such a way that it interferes with the uterine contractions that normally occur during menstruation, even the medical establishment acknowledges that this can cause menstrual cramps. There are a number of different gynecological conditions that can cause menstrual pain. The cramps are secondary to, or caused by, the underlying disease. These cramps are admitted to be not entirely in your head because the doctor can pinpoint a cause.

The other kind of menstrual pain, which is far more common, is primary dysmenorrhea. Primary dysmenorrhea is menstrual pain that is not known to be associated with a specific underlying disease. In other words, the doctor can't explain why you're having cramps. Primary dysmenorrhea is all in the woman's head, said most of the gynecology textbooks we had in medical school. Some of the texts would devote a couple of paragraphs to the notion that these cramps might be due to a hormone imbalance. Oh, they'd ob-

serve that women who, for one reason or another,
aren't ovulating—that is, they aren't releasing a ripe
egg from their ovaries each month and therefore
aren't producing certain hormones—rarely seemed to
have cramps, which indicates that cramps may be related to hormones. But that was generally about as
far as they'd go with that notion, before turning to
the more usual "psychogenic theory" of menstrual
cramps. *Psychogenic* means "of psychological origin."
In other words, it's back to the it's-all-in-your-head
theory that I'd first heard perpetrated by my gym
teacher, and had pretty much accepted ever since.

But now that I was having cramps myself, all that
went right out the window. These cramps were not in
my head! They were right there, in my belly, and they
hurt. I never have had really bad cramps, but these
were real enough to make me believe in other wom-
en's cramps. If I was having moderate cramps, then I
could certainly conceive of another woman having
mild ones and yet another having severe ones. Actually, I was always able to conceive of a woman having
cramps, even before I had them myself. I acknowledged the reality of the pain that women with primary dysmenorrhea experienced; I simply thought
the pain was psychogenic in origin.

If the consequences weren't so cruel, it would be almost comical to think back on the logic we used to
shore up our belief that a woman's pain was all in her
head. About ten to fifteen percent of women have
menstrual pain so severe that aspirin wouldn't handle it, and they're bothered enough to see the doctor.
These women were often distraught, high-strung,
nervous. We took this as evidence that they were neurotic types, given to psychosomatic ailments. We
thought their emotional state was the *cause* of their
pain. It didn't occur to us that maybe their emotional
state was the *result* of the pain.

I think part of the reason doctors persist in thinking

menstrual cramps are all in your head is that most doctors are men and have never themselves experienced cramps. Also, I think doctors don't like to admit the reality of something they can neither explain nor treat, so they have a tendency to turn the whole thing around, projecting it on to the patient: I can't find anything wrong with you, therefore you must be crazy.

The old it's-all-in-your-head-dearie diagnosis gets used a lot in gynecology. There's a general belief that women's pain is often unreal. I can remember how we'd talk about women who'd be complaining, moaning or even screaming during labor and childbirth. We'd often say to each other, "Oh, she's not really in that much pain." We'd go in and put our hands on the woman's belly and feel her uterus tightening up as she had a contraction. Sometimes you'd feel a woman's uterus and it would be tight and hard as a rock, but the woman wouldn't be having much pain. Then, you'd feel another woman's uterus and the contraction wouldn't be very hard at all, but she'd be screaming about the pain. In our minds, she was just making it up. If we couldn't feel her pain, then it wasn't real.

Almost every woman experiences menstrual cramps at some time or another in her life, yet medical science persists in saying that the pain is unreal, that it's psychosomatic. It might seem strange that the science of gynecology holds with the belief that half the human race is neurotic enough to experience psychosomatic pain, but this isn't so hard to understand if you look at what gynecologists are taught about the female personality. In medical school, we're taught that three traits compose the core of the female personality: feminine narcissism, feminine masochism, and feminine passivity. If one is taught to believe that women are masochists, it's not hard to adopt the view that their pain is not real.

It took me a number of years to see the connections between how doctors treated nurses, how women's pain is viewed by doctors, and what doctors are taught about the female personality. Once I began to make those connections, I would change the kind of doctor I was in very important ways, but that was still years away. Still, the day I had cramps myself made some real and immediate differences in how I treated my women patients and how I reacted to their pain, whether it was menstrual pain or some other kind.

Not long after my first bout with cramps, I saw a woman in clinic one afternoon who was a new subscriber to the medical plan for which my hospital was the central facility. I always tried to look over a patient's chart before I went in to examine her so I'd have some idea of what she was there for, whether it was a vaginal infection, contraception, a routine pelvic or whatever. All it said on this woman's chart under the "Reason for Seeking Appointment" heading was "referred by Psych." It wasn't all that uncommon for gynecology to refer a patient from our department to the psychology department for counseling, but I'd never seen it happen the other way around. I was curious.

The woman, who was sitting on the edge of the examining table, looked to be in her late twenties. She had straight dark hair and wore large glasses. There was a sensible, studious air about her; she looked normal enough. I guess, because she was a Psych referral, I had expected some disheveled maniac. (I did not have very enlightened attitudes about psychology either in those days.) She was very matter-of-fact, explaining that she had changed employers a few months ago, and so was now covered under our medical plan. She had been in psychotherapy for three years, and the cost of therapy had been a drain on her budget. When she found out that the medical plan offered therapy, she'd decided to switch. Besides, despite three years of psychotherapy, her problem wasn't getting any better. In fact it was getting worse. She had thought switching therapists might help. So far it hadn't.

The problem that led her to see a psychiatrist in the first place was that for the past six years severe, incapacitating pain accompanied her period. She would also get nauseated and vomit, and suffer violent diarrhea. She'd seen a number of gynecologists over the years, and none of them had been able to find anything physically wrong with her or to provide any relief for her symptoms. Her new psychiatrist had suggested she have yet another gynecological exam, so here she was.

I could tell she didn't have much hope that I was going to uncover a physical basis for her problem, and I didn't. I gave her a prescription for painkillers and something to control the vomiting and diarrhea. Normally, I'd just have sent her back to the psychiatrist with a note saying there didn't seem to be any physical cause for her symptoms; I guess it was my own recent bout with menstrual cramps that kept me from dismissing her accordingly. But beyond that, she didn't seem that neurotic to me. She was tense and nervous, but hell, I figured, if I'd been vomiting and having pain every month for six years, I'd probably be tense too.

I explained that I couldn't find anything wrong with her, but that I wanted to examine her when she was menstruating and was actually having the symptoms. So we arranged an appointment for the following week when her period was due to start.

Meanwhile I called over to Psych and made an appointment to see her psychiatrist to discuss her case. This was not something I would normally have done, because I thought psychiatry was another form of witchcraft. The nuttiest people in my medical school class were the ones who went into psychiatry. None-

theless, I went over to Psych to see her shrink who
turned out to be one of those people who wanted to
talk endlessly, perhaps because, being a shrink, he
spent all his time listening to other people. Now that
he had a chance to have someone listen to him, he
was going to take full advantage of it. Anyhow, he
went on for a good hour and a half about this woman's id and her ego and her superego and her Electra
complex and the other inflated jargon I thought all
psychiatrists used. What it boiled down to was this:
The woman's father had wanted a boy, so to please
her father and win his love and approval, she was at-
tempting to reject her femininity by becoming very
career-oriented, which caused her to throw up each
time she had her period.

Maybe, I cautioned myself, my reaction to what he
was saying was too flip and glib. Maybe this woman's
menstrual problems really were a manifestation of her
rejection of her own femininity. It's certainly possible
that someone could be that crazy. There are, after all,
mental institutions full of people who put cigarettes
out on themselves, think they're God, and in general
behave very strangely. But, the psychiatrist's analysis just did not have the ring of psychic truth. It
didn't jibe with what I'd seen of this woman. In fact I
thought it was all a crock of shit.

I asked him why he'd sent her to see me. He told
me that her "persistent fantasy that her problems had
a physical origin" was interfering with his attempts
to have her come to terms with the true origins of
her problem, so he wanted her to see a doctor who
would, once again, verify that there was nothing
physically wrong with her.

"Well, I can't say that. All I'm saying is that I
couldn't find anything. It's possible that there *is*
something physically wrong," I pointed out.

He gave me a condescending smile and told me that
it was very easy to get caught up in a patient's delu-

sional system, especially if one was not a trained psychiatrist like himself. I took my leave of him politely,
without saying anything about his own delusional
system.

I saw the woman again the following week. She
dragged herself into my office in a state of acute misery, and threw up twice during the exam. I did a very
thorough exam, but I still couldn't find anything
wrong. She was too sick for me even to talk to her, so
I asked her to come back in a few days when she was
feeling better. Meanwhile, I went to one of the surgeons I was assigned to at the time and explained the
situation to him. I told him I wanted to do an exploratory laparoscopy on her. In this procedure, a laparoscope, a tubular, periscope-type viewing instrument,
is inserted into the pelvic cavity through a small incision in the abdomen. It allows you to take a look-see
without actually cutting open the abdomen and going
into the pelvic cavity.

He agreed to see the woman. When she came back
the following week, I suggested the possibility of an
exploratory laparoscopy and, fed up with the pain
and uncertainty she'd been living with, she agreed.
So I sent her over to see the staff doctor. He too could
find no indication of anything physically wrong, but
agreed with me that the severity of her symptoms
warranted further investigation, and we scheduled
her for surgery.

I did the procedure myself, with the staff man assisting me. As soon as she was fully anesthetized, I
made the incision, put the laparoscope in, adjusted
the eyepiece, peered down into her pelvic cavity and
gave a long, low whistle.

"Look here," I told the staff doctor.

"My god," he said, "I've never seen one that bad
before."

The woman's entire pelvic cavity was studded with
tiny blueberrylike dots. She had an extensive case of

endometriosis, a condition in which little bits of endometrial tissue, the kind of tissue that lines the inside
of the uterus, are found growing outside the uterus.
Endometrial tissue is the part of the uterine lining that
thickens and swells each month in preparation for a
possible pregnancy. If pregnancy does not occur, the
endometrial lining breaks down and is shed in the
form of menstrual blood. Normally, endometrial tissue is only found on the inside of the uterus, but in
women with endometriosis, this tissue shows up in
other places. Just like the endometrial tissue inside
the uterus, these abnormally located bits of
endometrial tissue respond to the monthly ebb and
flow of hormones, and they too thicken and swell and
then break down each month. The problems occur because the lining of the pelvic cavity is extremely sensitive to blood, and when these bits of endometrial tissue start menstruating, all hell can break loose. If, as
had occurred in this woman, the bowels are involved,
there may be vomiting, diarrhea or constipation. The
condition can, indeed, be extremely painful.

It took us hours to clean out her pelvic cavity and
get rid of all those little bits of endometrial tissue.
Sometimes it's necessary to follow up the surgery
with drug therapy, but it wasn't in this woman's case.
I don't know if she ever got around to accepting whatever it was she'd been rejecting according to the smug
psychiatrist, but she did stop vomiting every time she
had her period, and the cramps and diarrhea disappeared. She came dancing into my office for her first
post-op visit and announced that she was having her
first pain-free menstrual period in six years and
wasn't so much as slightly nauseated.

Needless to say, she thought I was the greatest
thing since sliced bread. I rather thought so myself.
She couldn't thank me enough, and I loved it. This
business is not all bad.

FIVE

ANGING OUT with the nurses and dealing with women's pain as if it were real, as opposed to psychosomatic, were the beginnings of what would one day become a feminist viewpoint, but at that point in time, the early spring of 1967, I could hardly have been called a feminist. To me, all women's libbers were crazy ladies, like the ones I'd seen on the Johnny Carson show dressed up in Superman costumes—just another bunch of nuts.

Even so, I took a fair amount of ribbing from the other residents. "Hey, Jane, you're not getting into that women's libber stuff, are you? Not gonna go out and burn your bra, are you?" they'd leer.

They didn't have anything to worry about. As far as I could see, women's lib was for housewives who wanted to go out and get jobs or get their husbands to do the dishes. I had a job. I didn't have a husband. I did my own dishes. And why anyone would want to set fire to a perfectly good bra was beyond me. It seemed none of these things had relevance to my life.

Besides, women's libbers were for legalizing abortion. I had taken the Hippocratic Oath. I believed in that oath, and it specifically said, "Nor will I give a woman a pessary to procure abortion." For me, there was really no question about it, or if there were questions, I had the answers to them all: Abortion was legally and morally wrong.

It wasn't that I thought of abortion as killing, not exactly; I didn't think of a fetus as alive in the usual sense. All those religious arguments about when life begins and whether or not a fetus is alive have always seemed to me to be so much academic mumbo jumbo, about as meaningful as the debates of medieval theologians who sat around arguing about how many angels could sit on the head of a pin. I didn't and don't know when life, whatever that means, begins. Still, abortion went against the grain, and though I had never thought about it very seriously, my attitude was more than a mere rote catechism or a simple knee-jerk reaction conditioned by my upbringing and medical training. It went much deeper than that.

In part, my attitude towards abortion grew out of my profound respect for the incredibly intricate and beautiful process of conception. There is more here than the simple mechanics of an egg popping off the ovary and bumping into a sperm in the fallopian tube. First, there is the ovary, deep within the body, that, propelled by some unknown force, turns once a month towards the funnel-like opening at the end of the fallopian tube. On the surface of the ovary is a tiny bubble, a blister, that contains the one egg that alone, for some mysterious reason, has emerged from a field of two hundred and fifty thousand to ripen that month.

Suddenly the bubble bursts. Triggered by a surge of luteinizing hormone, an eloquent chemical messenger from the brain, the ovary contracts sharply and the ripe egg bursts forth. The fringed projections at the end of the fallopian tube reach out like fingers to grasp the ovum and draw it into the narrow tunnel of the tube. In a dreamlike, slow-motion ballet, thousands of tiny, undulating cilia caress the ripening egg and gently move it along on its four-inch, four-day journey to the womb.

At the same time, the microscopic sperm deposited in the vagina are making what is, considering their size, an impossibly long journey. Guided by a direction-finding mechanism whose nature we can only guess at, the sperm swim up the vagina, past the barrier of the cervix, into the womb itself. They must then navigate the entire length of the uterus and swim into the narrow upper reaches of the dark fallopian tube to meet and fertilize the egg.

The process is precisely orchestrated, the coordination of the myriad of biologic details staggeringly complex. It is, for instance, only at this time of the month, when a woman is ovulating, that mucus produced by the glands in her cervix will allow sperm to pass through the cervix and into the womb. At other times of the month, the molecules of the mucus form a crosshatched pattern to block the sperm lest they reach an egg too young or too old to be properly fertilized, thus producing a deformed baby. At the right moment, though, the molecules of the mucus realign themselves, forming microscopic tunnels to aid the sperm on their journey.

The biochemical communications system that orchestrates all this is so sophisticated that it makes the technology of beaming planetwide transmissions off orbiting satellites look like child's play. When the sperm finally meet the egg, they secrete a series of enzymes that soften the outer shell of the egg and make it permeable. Meanwhile, other chemicals secreted in the tube have completed the ripening of the egg so it is ready to accept the sperm that has managed to permeate the outer shell. The sperm and ovum lock genetic arms, a mating of a still more complex biochemistry, and the mingled DNA and RNA of the mother and father create a blueprint from which a unique human being will grow.

Once fertilized, the egg completes its journey down into the uterus. The uterus, notified of the impending pregnancy through an elaborate chemical communications system, has grown thick and rich. The blood vessels in the uterine lining flood the area with a rich supply of blood, and the uterine glands pour forth a banquet of nutrients for the developing egg. For the first three days after its arrival in the uterus, the tiny egg floats freely within the plush garden of the uterus. It implants in the uterine lining on the seventh day.

It takes, then, seven days to complete this journey—from the moment the egg bursts out of the ovary and begins to move through the darkness of the tube towards the possibility of the creation of life and the implantation of the fertilized egg in the uterus. It is a journey we all know; it is engraved upon our genetic memories and etched inside each tiny molecule of DNA in every cell in our bodies. It is a journey our species tells of over and over again in the ancient archetypal legends of heroic gods and goddesses who travel from darkness into light to be reborn, and in the primal myths of creation that form the basis of all our religions. It is the story of our personal and racial creation. It is, indeed, a holy story, and the entire process touches some deep chord in me. I have a profound respect for the beauty and delicate intricacy of it; its complexity humbles me. To interfere with this awesome process, to perform an abortion, was an unthinkably arrogant and wanton act. No. Abortion was wrong. Period. End of discussion.

That abortions were illegal did not, of course, stop women from having them, so even though we didn't do them ourselves, we spent a fair amount of time cleaning up after illegal abortion attempts. The most common problem attending illegal abortions was infection. Now that abortion has been legalized, severely infected abortions, known in medicalese as septic abortions, are a rarity, but back then they were so common that large hospitals would have wards devoted exclusively to them.

We used to refer to the septic abortion cases as

"Tijuana Specials." Women who were pregnant and didn't want to be would take weekend vacations across the border to Tijuana and other Mexican towns, where abortions were, if not legal, at least available. The trouble was that while these border towns had a certain quaint and dusty native charm, they weren't noted for their standards of cleanliness. If a woman was lucky, she might be able to find a skilled abortionist who had a fairly clean set-up. Not everyone was lucky. By Tuesday night, the unlucky ones would start coming into the emergency room, weak, faint, feverish, vomiting, in pain and sometimes bleeding.

Many of the Tijuana Specials we saw were undoubtedly performed here in the United States. If "Tijuana Special" has a callous ring to it, the term was, nonetheless, an accurate reflection of our attitudes towards the women who had them. First of all, we considered them a real pain; they kept the resident on duty up half the night. Each time a blood pressure dropped or a fever soared, the resident had to drag out of bed and order more intravenous antibiotics or whatever else the situation required. But it was more than simple crankiness about the inconvenience that accounted for our feelings. We had contempt for these women, who, we thought, had been stupid or irresponsible about birth control. After all, the great gods of medical technology had wrought wonders in the field of contraception, including the nearly perfect contraceptive, the Pill. If women would just take their Pills, then long-suffering residents wouldn't have to be kept up all night with their messy abortions.

If we'd sat down and thought about it, we'd have realized how unfair this point of view was. Not all women—least of all, young teenagers—had access to the Pill, and many of those who did were reluctant to use it because of their fear of side effects—which, as it would eventually turn out, was not an unwarranted fear. Moreover, the available methods of birth control were only about ninety-eight percent effective. This means that in a group of one hundred women using that method for a year, ninety-eight wouldn't get pregnant, but two would. But that's only for one year. Women have about thirty-five fertile years in their lifetimes. A rate of two unplanned pregnancies per year over a period of thirty-five years could mean some seventy unwanted pregnancies in a group of one hundred women. So even if a woman dutifully swallows her Pills, uses her diaphragm or whatever, the odds are that she may still face an unwanted pregnancy at some time in her life.

But we didn't think about that. Even if we had thought about it, the prevailing medical and social ethic held that a woman who got pregnant was supposed to have the baby, regardless. The implications of this moral principle in terms of the population crisis was something else we conveniently didn't think about, at least not then.

A free-floating moral hypocrisy also colored our attitude toward these women. Many of them were unmarried, and the so-called sexual revolution had as yet only the most tremulous toehold on American mores. Nice girls didn't do it. These girls had obviously done it; therefore they were not nice girls. Unwanted pregnancy was considered just punishment for the sin of premarital sex. They could hardly expect to have their cake and eat it too. Never mind that many of the doctors were unmarried and had cake crumbs on their lips. That was something else we conveniently didn't think about. On the other hand, we felt no more sympathy for the married woman who sought abortion. *That* was worse than not liking apple pie, a real slap in the face of American motherhood.

One Tuesday evening in April of sixty-seven, a

sixteen-year-old girl came into ER. She was running a fever and had pains in her lower abdomen. Her blood pressure was low, only 80 over 60. I was on call in Gynecology, and they asked me to come down to ER and do a pelvic exam on her.

I spoke briefly with the nurse who'd admitted the girl and went in to see her. I found her curled up on the examining room table.

"What's been the problem?" I asked. She was groggy, which wasn't surprising considering her blood pressure. Talking to her was difficult. Her responses were slow and her voice so faint that I could hardly catch her words, but I managed to find out that she'd been running a fever for a couple of days, vomiting off and on, and had cramps—bad ones that kept getting worse. When she'd gotten up to go to the bathroom, she'd fainted, so her mother brought her into the hospital.

I asked when she'd had her last period and whether she'd ever been pregnant. She told me that her last period had been a couple of weeks ago and no, she'd never been pregnant. I got the nurse who'd admitted the girl to come in and assist with the pelvic exam. The girl's uterus was enlarged and exquisitely tender. Her cervix was slightly lacerated. The cervical os, the opening to the uterus, was dilated, and I could see that some of the products of conception were still inside her badly infected uterus. Another Tijuana Special. I finished the exam, got her out of the stirrups and tried to put some gentleness into my voice.

"Look," I said, "I know that you've had an abortion, and in order to take care of you properly I need to know when it was done and what was used."

She didn't want to cooperate with me. She insisted that she couldn't possibly be pregnant; she hadn't had an abortion.

I don't know what abortionists used to tell their clients (maybe that they too would go to jail), but almost always, no matter how badly they'd been butchered, no matter what kind of pain they were in, even if they were bleeding all over the place, patients maintained a bizarre loyalty to the abortionist. It was as if the abortionists were the good guys and we were the bad guys. It would be a number of years before I would begin to see that they had a point.

I explained to the girl that the abortion was incomplete, that she had a massive infection and that I was going to have to admit her and clean out her uterus. A little "Okay," which sounded like it came from someplace far away, was all I got in reply. I ordered intravenous antibiotics and the necessary pre-op tests. I told the nurse to prep her and get her upstairs to the operating room, and I went out to talk to the mother.

It was now about one in the morning, and the waiting room was empty except for a thin, birdlike woman perched on the edge of a chair. She sat very straight, her body stiffly erect, knees close together. The knuckles on the hands that clutched the purse in her lap were white. She was a worn, worried woman.

"Mrs. Boggs?" I introduced myself, "I'm Dr. Patterson."

"Is my little girl all right?" she broke in anxiously.

I guessed that a woman who called her daughter "my little girl" wouldn't know anything about the pregnancy or the abortion. I didn't like telling her, but I had no choice. I needed her permission in order to admit the girl. There was also an outside chance that she might have known how the bungled procedure had been done, what had been used. At the least, she should be able to give me some idea of when it was done.

I explained the situation to the mother. Though what I was telling her came as a shock, her first concern was her daughter's health. She was willing to cooperate with me, but she knew nothing about the abortion attempt. She told me that her daughter had gone down to San Diego on Friday to visit a girlfriend and hadn't been feeling well when she came home Sunday night. I guessed that the daughter had had the abortion on Saturday or, possibly, on Sunday. I explained that I was going to have to take her daughter into the operating room. She asked if she could see the girl first, and I took her back to the examining room.

The nurse had set up the IV, and the technician was drawing blood when we came into the room. The girl, her hair tucked up into a green surgical cap, looked even younger than her sixteen years. She turned her head towards us as we came into the room and cried, "Mommy!" The mother wove her way between the nurse, the IV, and all the other paraphernalia, to her daughter's side and kissed her forehead.

"I'm sorry, Mommy," the girl said.

"It's okay, baby. It's okay," the mother told her. "You could have told me, honey. It's okay, don't you worry about it now. You just get better."

The mother stood there, wiping her daughter's brow and making the cooing sounds mothers make to comfort their sick kids. I left them there and went upstairs to scrub up.

The D&C—the dilation and curettage, the procedure used to empty the uterus—went fairly smoothly. The girl lost a good deal of blood and needed a transfusion, but although her blood pressure was low, it was holding. I took her to the recovery room, checked her out and left orders for the nurse to monitor her and call me if things got any worse.

By this time I was thoroughly exhausted. I went up to the on-call room and fell asleep. Within what seemed like only a few minutes, the phone rang. It was a STAT call, a medical emergency: The girl was in trouble. I took the staircase three steps at a time. The anesthesiologist must have taken them four at a time, because he was already in her room when I got there. As I came through the door, I glanced at the EKG. It had gone flat. The girl's heart had stopped.

The anesthesiologist started working her chest, rhythmically pumping. He cracked a rib and swore softly. "Forget it," I told him. A cracked rib was the least of the girl's problems.

The anesthesiologist worked on her for a few more minutes, then motioned for me to take over. Pumping somebody's heart is hard work. We alternated, taking turns rhythmically pushing on her chest. We continued spelling each other, anxiously watching the clock. Too many minutes were going by. He took over, and I checked the EKG, which was still flat. I stood there holding one of her limp hands, but she didn't know it. She wasn't breathing on her own, and she wasn't going to. We all knew it and had known it for twenty minutes, but it was hard to quit hoping. Finally, the anesthesiologist said, "I think this is useless." He was right. We pronounced the girl dead at 3:45 AM.

I went down to the waiting room to tell the mother. She was perched in the same spot, but now her hands were clutching another set of hands instead of her purse. This set of hands belonged to a woman with a long, gentle face. I was glad there was someone else there.

I told the mother, as softly as you can tell such hard news, that her daughter was dead. A tiny, wounded noise came out of her mouth. For a few moments, she didn't change her expression or move her lips. Then she buried her head in the other woman's chest and sobbed, that terrible dry kind of sobbing that makes no noise. The other woman, who turned out to be the girl's aunt, sort of curled around the mother and held her tight, rocking her back and forth and making vague, comforting noises. We all sat there for a while, silent. There was nothing to say.

"I'm sorry," I said.

The girl's aunt began to talk, thanking me, reassuring me. I'd done my best, all that was possible, she said; this wasn't my fault. She talked on, about making "the arrangements." It was okay, she would take care of things; she always had. She talked about her sister's girl, about how she was such a good girl, really. She began to babble her memories, and soon she was crying.

"Why?" she asked no one in particular. "Why did this have to happen?"

I no longer had all the answers. Maybe abortion was a crime, but being sixteen years old and pregnant and scared and trying to get an abortion isn't criminal, it's sad. And even if it was a crime, the punishment didn't fit the crime. The girl didn't *deserve* to die. No sixteen-year-old kid *deserves* to die.

The aunt sat there, saying it over and over again: "Why did this have to happen?"

No, I no longer had all the answers.

SIX

I HAD no answers for the aunt, and, worse, none for myself.

What I did have was a complex and almost unbearable grief, and a terrible, sharp ache in my throat. But, having learned what I thought was my lesson with the Harts, I was properly professional and dry-eyed. With an iron effort, I managed to go on about my business that night acting as if the world were actually an okay place to live in. Finally, I made it back to the on-call room, and then, as I closed the door safely behind me, there she was again, the Lady of the Lake, who, despite all my eviction notices, still lived at the center of me, and I cried and cried and cried.

The crying was, as always, overwhelming. It was the kind of crying that people who cannot allow themselves to feel much of their pain do when it finally becomes too much to sit on anymore. It came tearing out of me with the energy of big things kept too long in small, tight places. It came out in great, powerful waves.

I cried for the mother, for that worn-out looking woman with the indelible stamp of women who scrape along at the edge of life, working some dreary job year in and out, sustained only by the dream of giving their children a chance at something better than they themselves have had. I wept, seeing her again huddled against her sister there in the waiting room, broken, her last light gone out, all her years of caring and sacrifice, of making do—all that love extinguished with the death of her daughter.

I wept for the daughter too. She was just a kid. She should have been home, posing in front of mirrors, making herself up as young girls do, imagining a life of impossible glamour, getting ready to go out into the world and make of herself, for ill or good, what she would. She shouldn't be lying there, the life torn out of her.

As usual, once I was forced into the luxury of tears, my crying was about much more than the incident that provoked it. This time it was not about one child's death, but about all the women I'd seen who had died or been maimed or crippled or made less than whole in what we called the septic tank. It was about the terrible injustice and meanness of life that is more than any of us should have to bear. The tears were also for myself, for my having to stand there helplessly, a young girl's hand in mine, while the life flowed out of her. And, ultimately, I was crying for the loss of my simple certainties, for the loss of the black and white rules by which I'd lived my life, rules that had suddenly gone all grey.

"Why did this have to happen?" the aunt had wanted to know, and the answer, of course, was that it *didn't* have to happen. The girl could have had an abortion in a safe, clean place—a properly sterilized hospital operating room—instead of some godawful back alley. If my commitment was to saving lives, what about the girl's life? Why should the life of a clump of insensate cells a few weeks old take precedence over the life of a living, breathing, feeling human being? And now, because of this child's death, I found myself facing a more terrible question: By denying women access to abortions, was the medical profession saving lives or taking them?

I now felt it was wrong to deny women abortions;

still, when women came to me seeking abortions, I refused, though my refusal no longer had the frosty ring of moral superiority—not that this mattered much to those poor, desperate women. I justified my refusal by reminding myself of the illegality of the procedure and telling myself that abortion was medically dangerous. Didn't I have ample proof of this in the flood of septic abortions we treated? Of course, I knew I was seeing only the one in a hundred or the one in a thousand or, who knows, the one in ten thousand, who ran into trouble.

My belief that abortion was dangerous conveniently allowed me to sidestep my conscience. I clung to it because I simply wasn't willing to put my career on the line. Performing abortions, or even referring women to another doctor who would, could have meant losing my medical license or going to jail. I had too much invested in my career to do that.

I don't know how long I would have gone on tap dancing around the issue. I like to think it wouldn't have been forever, but any soul searching I might eventually have gotten around to was short-circuited by Ronald Reagan. In June 1967, barely two months after the girl's death, Reagan, then governor of California, signed into law a bill that allowed doctors to perform abortions if the mother's physical or mental condition was such that continuing the pregnancy would endanger her life. There was nothing new in allowing doctors to perform abortions in those rare medical instances in which the mother's physical state was so precarious that carrying a pregnancy to term would have killed her; but there was something very new indeed in allowing the mother's mental condition to be considered in the abortion decision. Under the terms of this new law, a woman could get an abortion if she could find, and afford to pay, two pyschiatrists who were willing to say that she was suicidally depressed over the pregnancy and might take her own life if the pregnancy was not terminated.

I suppose that I should have known that such a change in the law was in the works, but my life was lived with my nose so close to the grindstone that I saw events outside the walls of the hospital with myopic vision, dim and blurred. And even if my sight had been more acute, it would never have occurred to me that Ronald Reagan, the darling of the arch-conservatives, the home-and-family, mom-and-apple-pie traditionalist, would have signed a liberalized abortion law that was so much at odds with his political persona. This was pre-Watergate America: We were, most of us, still naive enough to expect some sort of connection between our politicians' rhetoric and their political actions. (Reagan later claimed that he did not understand the implications of the California Therapeutic Abortion Act of 1967. I don't know what disturbs me more—his anti-abortion stance or the fact that this man, now the president of our nation, may still be signing bills whose implications he doesn't fully grasp.)

At any rate, the new law took me completely by surprise, and I had lots of company. As soon as the law was passed, there was a virtual epidemic of suicidal depression among pregnant women in the state of California. Women began pouring into hospitals, clinics and doctors' offices throughout the state. We were in no way prepared to deal with them. The hospital bureaucracy, like all large and lumbering beasts, was not equipped to move quickly. But in this case there was no choice. You can't tell a woman seeking an abortion to please come back in a month, after you've had time to create a new batch of forms in triplicate and enough red tape to deal with the situation. The longer a pregnancy continues, the more dangerous it is to abort, until, if you've waited too long, it is no longer possible to do the abortion at all.

The hospital bureaucracy responded with unaccustomed agility. The law was passed on a Tuesday, as I recall, and by Thursday the chief had held an emergency department meeting to explain the new law to us. He emphasized that doing abortions was a matter of personal choice and that anyone who had personal or religious objections wouldn't be expected to perform them. I think many of the staff had the same ambivalence about abortion that I had, but they too had seen the horrors of the septic tank, women dying at the hands of back alley abortionists, women dead from trying to flush their insides out with lye, women maimed and crippled for life. Like me, they were thankful for some way out.

And the new law afforded some protection for our consciences. After all, we had two psychiatric reports saying that there was a good chance this woman was going to commit suicide—an act that would have killed the fetus in any case. We heard through the hospital grapevine, which was always on full buzz, that a couple of doctors on the OB/GYN staff had refused, but for the most part, the staff signed on.

Under the new law, the two psychiatric evaluations, along with a gynecologist's report confirming the woman's pregnancy, were reviewed by an abortion review committee and the request for an abortion was either approved or disapproved. The hospital didn't have an abortion review committee, but this problem was solved in one neat bureaucratic stroke: The name of the Sterilization Review Committee, which approved requests for sterilization was changed to the Sterilization and Abortion Review Committee, and all the new paperwork was dumped on the renamed committee. The psychiatric evaluations were a bit of a joke. Only a few changes in phrasing or vocabulary kept them from being identical copies of each other. Most of the psychiatrists probably felt that if a woman said she was considering suicide because of an unwanted pregnancy, who were they to say she wouldn't actually do it? No one wanted to be in the position of writing an evaluation saying the woman wasn't really suicidal and then receiving a call from Emergency one night saying that the patient had been brought in dead or dying. Then too, like those of us on the GYN staff, the Psych staff had seen the tragic results of unwanted pregnancies and were glad to have some way to help these women.

Within a week of the passage of the new law, we were doing our first abortions. In those days we performed abortions on women in the first trimester (the first twelve weeks) of pregnancy by doing a dilation and curettage, a D&C. A D&C is a fairly simple procedure that involves knocking a woman out with a general anesthetic and gently dilating the cervical canal (the opening that leads from the vagina through the cervix and into the uterus) with a series of dilating rods of gradually increasing diameter. Once the cervix is sufficiently dilated, we used a curette, a sharp spoonlike instrument, to remove the contents of the uterus. It was a routine procedure used to diagnose and treat women with prolonged and excessive menstrual periods, uterine cancer, septic abortions or incomplete miscarriages, and we were all familiar with it.

I scrubbed on the morning of my first abortion, and perhaps I scrubbed a little longer than usual. Maybe I wanted to be extra careful about the possibility of infection, having seen so many septic cases, or maybe I was trying to delay doing what I had to do.

I had told myself that doing an abortion wouldn't be much different from doing a D&C on a woman who'd had an incomplete miscarriage. But it was different. For one thing, it was much bloodier. I am a surgeon. I am used to blood and pus and piss and all the outpourings of the human body. It is part of the daily business of my life. It should not have bothered me that it was so bloody. There is always a good deal of blood with a D&C; it's to be expected. But with an incomplete miscarriage, most of the blood and tissue have been expelled during the miscarriage. We have to deal only with what the body is unable to rid itself of. I was not prepared for blood lying in great, red puddles on the floor, and perhaps the blood seemed even more copious than it was because I was so reluctant to pass the sharp edged curette into the womb and cut away at what lay within.

At first it was not so bad. The women I operated on were only about eight weeks pregnant. At eight weeks the fetus is less than an inch long, smaller than your thumb. It has arms and legs and even the beginnings of separate little fingers and toes, but in the bloody soup of cut-up tissue spooned out of the womb, it's impossible to distinguish anything even vaguely recognizable as a fetus.

Then, a few weeks after the law was passed, I aborted a woman who was twelve weeks pregnant. The chief was assisting me. The woman we were operating on was one of his patients, not anyone I knew. I think not knowing her made it harder for me. If I had known her personally, I might have seen and felt things more completely from her point of view, which in turn might have made what happened in the operating room easier for me to deal with.

Aborting a twelve-week pregnancy is technically more difficult than aborting an earlier pregnancy. In fact, twelve weeks is the maximum for aborting a pregnancy by D&C. The cervix can be dilated manually only to a certain point. Opening it up further would damage the cervix, and after twelve weeks the fetus is over three and a half inches—too large to pass through a manually dilated cervical canal. I was very careful as I dilated her to this maximum point. I took it really slow.

Finally, I had the cervix sufficiently dilated, and I took the curette and began spooning out the contents of the uterus. The uterus is not a large organ. In women who are not pregnant, it's only about the size of a clenched fist. But the curette spoon is tiny, small enough to fit through the opening of the cervix, which, even when it's as widely dilated as it was in this woman, is only about twelve millimeters wide.

Emptying out the uterus with this tiny instrument is a tedious process. It takes a good five or ten minutes of spooning to empty out a nonpregnant uterus. When you're working on a pregnant woman, you have to remove not only the menstrual lining of the uterus, but also all the products of conception.

I had deposited about a dozen spoonfuls of bloody tissue into the metallic basin at my side. Although this was a good deal bloodier than doing an eight-week pregnancy and I could see that it was going to take longer, it wasn't really much different from the other abortions I'd been doing every Saturday morning for the past few weeks.

I carefully edged the curette through the passage I'd dilated in the cervix, angling for the next spoonful. As I was drawing the curette back out, I could feel a slight resistance as I pulled it into the cervical canal. This happens sometimes; you will snag on the edge of the curette a piece of tissue larger than the hollow of the spoon, and when you pull the instrument out through the canal, you feel resistance as the spongy tissue compresses into the canal. I tugged ever so gently, and the curette popped out of the cervix.

I stared, at first not comprehending, not wanting to comprehend, what I was seeing. Speared on the sharp cutting edge of the curette was a tiny leg.

The chief must have felt the shudder of revulsion that swept over me.

"With more advanced pregnancies, after about nine weeks, you're going to find that there will be identifiable portions of the conceptus in the material you're removing,'' the chief said in a dry, matter-of-fact, medical sort of way.

In my mind's eye I was traveling along the delicate slope of the ankle where the leg curves out into the foot, down to the five distinct, dainty, oh-so-tiny toes, when the chief's words caught me and brought my world, whose dimensions had momentarily gone all out of proportion, back into perspective. What he was saying was merely a fact. The world is an ordinary place: This was only another piece of medical data: After nine weeks, there are recognizable fetal parts in the material removed from the uterus. Yes, of course. It was all right, then. Facts I could handle. I knew what to do with facts; they were to be stored in the medical library in my mind along with the rest of my self-defensive armada of facts. This was a fact. It could be said out loud in words. In a sentence. It made sense. It was, after all, rational. Dealing with it as an objective fact made it possible to ward off the horror that was creeping in around the rational edges and to go on with the work at hand.

I held the curette over the basin. I tapped the stem of the curette on the metal lip of the bowl to empty the spoon. The tiny leg fell into the bowl with a soft plop that echoed about an operating room grown strangely quiet.

I worked in silence, removing more of the tissue, another tiny leg, two arms, a piecemeal torso. The bloody sludge in the metal basin grew more grotesque.

Finally, it seemed that I had finished. I stopped for a moment, setting the curette aside. With one hand pushing up on the uterus from inside and the other pressing down on the woman's abdomen, I outlined the contours of her uterus. It was smaller now, back to its normal size, indicating that it was empty. I took up a curette again and systematically moved it over the entire interior surface of the uterus. I closed my eyes, concentrating intensely while I made this final sweep, for if the uterus is indeed emptied, you will not feel any soft, spongy tissue, only the scrape of the curette on the hard muscle wall of the uterus. I brought my head down closer, turning it to one side as I worked, the better to hear, for if the uterus is emptied of all the soft tissue, you can hear the sound of the curette scraping along the muscle. This sound is called "the uterine cry." At that moment, the term seemed horribly apt.

The curette cried along the entire interior surface of her uterus. I felt no soft tissue, only firm muscle.

"I think that's it," I announced, opening my eyes and straightening up.

"Before you call it quits in this kind of situation," the chief said, "it's a good idea to double-check yourself, Jane. You've got the evacuated material here," he said, nodding towards the basin at my side, "and by examining it, you can make a better evaluation as to whether you've entirely evacuated the uterus."

What he was saying just would not register. I must have looked blank.

"See," he said, and picking up one of the discarded dilators, he began poking around in the contents of the bowl. The side of my body closer to the bowl went rigid and I arched slightly away, but my eyes were riveted on the bowl. I watched with a numb intensity as he separated the bloody hunks of tissue, pushing some aside and drawing others to the center of the bowl. With a few deft movements, he manipulated the tiny arms and legs and piecemeal torso into position. He tilted the bowl so the blood pooled in the lower edge of the basin, more clearly revealing the grisly jigsaw puzzle he'd assembled.

"I don't think you've got the head here," he said, sorting again through the tissue he had pushed aside.

"I think you've missed the head. Maybe not. It's hard to tell, but I think you'd better recheck it."

With something thick and tight at the center of me, I took another sterile curette from the scrub nurse and reached again into the uterus, feeling for any soft tissue that might still be floating around in the small hollow between the uterine walls.

The temperature in operating rooms is always on the cool side, but despite the chill, little rivers of perspiration trickled from the undersides of my breasts and down my arms.

I groped about in the hollow of the uterus.

"Yes, there is something," I said, striving for the properly detached tone as I rotated the curette in order to catch the piece of spongy tissue I had trapped between the spoon's underside and the uterine wall. Gingerly, I retracted the curette, but I lost the tissue. A nurse wiped the beads of sweat off my brow and I fished around again.

I caught it again and lost it again and swore under my breath. It took four tries before I managed to snag it and pull the tiny head, slightly larger than a nickel, through the dilated cervix. The baby's head—for now it was to me a baby, not a fetus—came out in a single piece. The jigsaw puzzle was complete, the procedure was over. I finished up in OR, changed out of my scrub suit, went into the bathroom and vomited.

I woke up at night for weeks afterwards, chased out of my sleep by nightmares whose dim shapes I could only vaguely recall.

It was only a few bare weeks after that abortion that I did my first amniocentesis abortion. In amniocentesis a hollow needle is inserted through the abdominal wall into the uterus and then into the sac of amniotic fluid that surrounds the developing fetus. Amniocentesis can be used to rule out the possibility of certain birth defects. It can also be used to abort. For the latter purpose, some of the fluid is drained from the sac and replaced with a solution of saline, which kills the fetus. Within twenty-four to thirty-six hours, the cervix dilates and the woman goes into labor and delivers the dead fetus.

At that time, this was the procedure we used to abort pregnancies that had progressed beyond the twelve-week point; however, the procedure was not done before sixteen weeks. There isn't enough fluid in the amniotic sac until then, and the danger of missing the sac and injecting the saline into a blood vessel is too great. Even at sixteen weeks, there is still a danger of hitting a blood vessel, which can have fatal consequences. For this reason, we don't anesthetize a woman undergoing the procedure. She needs to be aware, so she can tell us if she experiences any feeling of warmth, numbness, restlessness or headache—indications that saline has gotten into the bloodstream.

The woman on whom I was to perform my first amniocentesis was young, in her early twenties. She was lying on the cold metallic table; she said nothing, just lay there, her wide staring eyes focused on some distant point. I positioned a rack, something like a towel rack, below her breasts and above the rise of her belly, draping a surgical linen over it to block her view. Better that she not see what we were about to do. I swabbed her belly, once, twice, three times, with an antiseptic solution that stained her skin an unnatural reddish brown.

Now the needle, a shot of local anesthetic.

"You'll feel a slight prick, maybe a sensation of burning for a couple of seconds," I warned her.

She drew a deep, sharp breath.

I waited a bit, giving the anesthesia time to work. Then, I took the hollow amniocentesis needle from the tray and pressed it into her anesthetized skin. A thin, watery trickle of blood ran down her belly. I applied pressure to the needle, feeling it move through the layers of muscle and fat tissue and into the uterine wall.

"I think we're in," I said, meaning that the needle had pierced the uterine wall and was inside the sac. I held the needle steady as we threaded a length of transparent plastic tubing through the hollow of the needle. I breathed a sigh of relief as the clear amniotic fluid ran out of the tubing. No blood here. It appeared I hadn't hit a blood vessel. I let a sufficient quantity of fluid drain, and then, while I still held the needle, we hooked the tubing to the bottle of saline and the salt water began to flow down the tube. I took my hand off the needle and turned to the woman. If we'd somehow hit a blood vessel, we'd know now, from her reaction.

"Feeling okay?" I asked. She made a little sound of affirmation. "No headache, numbness, feeling of warmth, nausea?" No, she was fine.

Out of the corner of my eye I saw, or maybe just sensed, a movement. Startled, I turned to look. It was the needle. The needle was moving. I looked around thinking the nurse or the staff doctor had jarred the tube or bottle, but there was nobody near, and the needle was still wobbling back and forth, jerking this way and that as if something was knocking against it. Something, or, oh my god, somebody.

I lifted my eyes and looked across the table into the staff doctor's eyes, which fluttered shut and open again, confirming what I was seeing and thinking.

"It's a reflex," he said softly. "Just a reflex."

I wanted to be able to believe that.

The woman moaned.

"Are you all right, feeling any pain, nausea . . ." I reeled off my litany.

"No, no nothing like that . . ." Her voice trailed off and came back louder and hysterical around the edges.

"My baby, my baby . . . oh, my baby!"

Her voice had, for me, a tone of accusation, as if all this had nothing to do with her, but was some hideous crime I was inflicting on her. I was blindly furious, taking the jungle of emotion inside me and projecting it outward in anger at her. I wanted to scream, "Don't blame me, lady. I didn't put you here on this table. I didn't knock you up. Nobody's making you do this. It's *you* who are making *me* do it. This is your fault, not mine"—as if there were a fault here. I didn't, of course, say any of these things; I finished up, removing the tube, tight-lipped and stonily polite. It was not my finest moment as a physician.

The shape of the nightmares that woke me trembling in the middle of the night grew clearer. I woke with the taste of blood in the back of my mouth. What I was doing was murder, a cutting up of life. I sat for long hours in the close and private darkness, arguing with myself. I told myself that we are living on a lifeboat, a small planet sailing through a finite galaxy. There is just so much room in the lifeboat, and if we are not careful, there will not be enough room for all of us. Already there is not enough food. Children are dying, starving to death each minute, each second. We need to make some tough choices and we must make them now, before the lifeboat, overburdened, sinks.

And what of my more familiar debating point—the one about the rights of women to control their own reproductive organs?

I lay awake in those small hours of the morning making intellectual arguments with myself, but the real argument proceeded on an entirely different level. I was stretched thin and taut between two poles.

At one pole there was the tiny leg impaled on the curette, the moving needle, and the horror and revulsion I felt on a gut level. And deeper than even that personal experience, there was the primitive, insistent beat of the basic evolutionary imperative: Take care of the little ones. It's about survival. No species evolves without the compelling urge coded into the genes of all its individuals: Protect the young. And thus we are inevitably troubled by the thought of abortion.

At the other pole was the feel of that young girl's hand limp in mine as she lay there dying, her last light extinguished too soon.

I wanted no part of this. I wanted my world back the way it was, with its simple certainties and its neat rules. I wanted to go to the chief and tell him that I wanted none of this abortion business. Let someone else do it. But I could not. The jackboots of reality had come stomping through my smug little moral world, and the memory of the death of that sixteen-year-old girl was too insistent.

I know that those opposed to abortion say that, if we allow killing in the womb, then the next step, made in the name of necessity, will be killing the old or the enfeebled. I understand their fear. Since the time of Hippocrates, doctors have been sworn a solemn oath not to take life, not even when it would be merciful to end the painful last throes of the terminally ill. We have sworn that oath and kept to it because we know that putting the decision concerning death into human hands could lead to all manner of horrors. Such power could be too easily abused. Human hands cannot be relied upon to carry the burden of such life and death decisions; they are not strong enough.

And now, by permitting abortion, we are crossing a centuries-old line. But it is because of the eventual possibility of euthanasia for the elderly or feeble that we need now to cross that line, for if we do not, we will pass on to our children's children a world so overpopulated that such terrors might come to pass.

At that time I made what was possibly my first real

moral decision. I say my first because I don't count the situations in which there is a clear line between right and wrong. It is choosing between the not clearly right and the not clearly wrong, threading one's way through all the ambiguous grey areas, that constitutes a true moral decision.

In time, I made peace with myself and my nightmares passed. I have continued and will continue to do abortions. It is, I believe, a necessary and ultimately a moral choice in our age. I have come to believe that a woman's right to control her own reproductive organs supersedes whatever rights might be accorded the fetus.

Still, the ambivalence remains. A few years ago another method of abortion, called dilation and evacuation, or D&E, was developed. The D&E can be done from twelve to twenty weeks, so there is no longer any need to wait until sixteen weeks, when an amniocentesis abortion can be done. When the Center for Disease Control in Atlanta came out with definitive studies showing that the D&E was safer than amniocentesis, I decided to learn the procedure. I arranged to observe a D&E being done on a woman nineteen weeks pregnant. At nineteen weeks the fetus is significantly more developed than it is at twelve weeks. Standing there, watching as the fetus was extracted piece by piece, was more than I could handle.

I don't do D&E's. I do abortions up to twelve weeks. If a woman twelve to twenty weeks comes in, I refer her to an excellent clinic in the area. Past twenty weeks, up to twenty-four weeks (the legal limit for performing abortions), I will do amniocentesis abortions. There is nothing rational about not doing D&E's, when I will do amnios, but that's where I am. It doesn't make perfect sense. But what in life does?

SEVEN

I WENT to bed on the evening of June thirtieth, 1967, a very tired second-year resident. I woke up the next morning early enough to have time for a leisurely walk from my apartment to the hospital, before I began my third year of residency.

My apartment was conveniently near the hospital, in a neighborhood that had been the victim of rapid growth and feeble zoning. Once it had been a neighborhood of distinction, located on what were then the outskirts of Hollywood. Stately, if pretentious, homes of silent screen stars had lined the streets, set back from the rows of palm trees at curbside by circular drives, manicured hedges and improbably green lawns. The mansions gave way in the early fifties to apartment buildings of the glitter-impregnated, pink stucco, box variety, adorned by orange-billed, white wrought iron flamingoes set out to graze on the more modest lawns of this neighborhood in transition. Still, such architecture passing for glamour in the Hollywood of the fifties, the neighborhood remained for some time an acceptable, even classy address, home to Hollywood's young up-and-comers. But in the intervening fifteen or so years, the up-and-comers had up and gone, into the hills and canyons, leaving the flatlands, the chipped stucco, and the fading, peeling flamingoes to the down-and-outers—starving students, out of work actors, winos and hippies, all the assorted flotsam and jetsam of the urban tide.

Nothing remained of the area's former glory except the towering palms, which housed amid their untrimmed, dead fronds the neighborhood's considerable rat population. You could hear them at night scurrying around in the dead fronds and might have been able to pretend it was something more poetic, perhaps a gentle breeze rustling through the fronds, except that late at night you could see the rats jumping from tree to tree. Occasionally one would fall out of the palms, thudding on the walk before your feet, and once, to everyone's horror, right on a neighbor's head. I was thinking of moving.

As I walked along, I was mentally refiguring my meager budget, which, as of July first, that very day, had an extra fifty dollars in it because my salary was about to jump from three hundred and fifty dollars a month to the munificent sum of four hundred per (alas, before taxes). This new affluence was the result of my having been transformed, overnight, from a mere second-year resident into a third-year resident, a *senior* resident, and more than that, *the* Chief Resident on the Complicated Obstetrics ward. But by the end of my calculations, I had come to the conclusion that even as chief resident I'd have to dwell among the rats.

Still, despite my realization that I would not yet be living in splendor, I felt overwhelmed by my new title, and the responsibilities accruing to the job, of chief resident. No longer would one of the staff doctors or the chief be hovering reassuringly over my shoulder on each and every case. They would not be there at my elbow in OR, ready to seize the scalpel and to bail me out if I ran into trouble. That I'd been operating competently for months without their having to lift a finger was an irrelevant detail that morning. As of that day, or so it seemed to me, the buck stopped here.

I had just been transported to an entirely new level

of responsibility, only I didn't feel transformed. I felt panic, the same panic with which I'd greeted my first day on the wards as a medical student, my first day of internship, my first day of residency. There ought to be some rites of passage to mark your movement through each successive phase of a medical education, some ceremony that would affirm your new competence, helping create the confidence that in me at least was always lacking. But, there isn't.

I arrived at the hospital that morning in a state of composure akin to that of a young bird just nudged out of the nest for its first flight; I was inwardly squawking in terror. But I managed my usual "hey, everything's perfectly fine" masquerade, and much to my amazement, in the weeks that followed, I flew and flew smoothly.

When I first became an intern and found that a couple of months had gone by and I hadn't killed anyone, I began to develop a cocky self-assurance, and so it was during my first rotation as chief resident on Comp OB. By the time I'd finished my three months there and had gone on to become chief resident on Gynecological Surgery, I was fairly soaring. I had, in fact, begun to develop a rather exaggerated notion of my competence, which isn't hard if you're a doctor.

You arrive on the ward each morning, decked out in your magic cloak of authority (your white physician's coat), with your royal scepter (your stethoscope) slung importantly about your neck, or dangling conspicuously from your pocket. All the royal minions—the nurses, lab techs, orderlies, and patients—address you by title, "Yes, Doctor," "Right away, Doctor." You, on the other hand, speaking with, at best, the graciousness of a Southern plantation owner, address the field hands on a first-name basis, or if you are so arrogant and self-important that you haven't even bothered to learn their names, as "dearie" or "honey" or "you there" or by function,

as in "Nurse, get me this," "Orderly, do that." And
there are few, if any, who question your royal prerogatives. You develop a certain swagger and go strut-
ting pompously about, and rather than laughing
outright or giggling behind your back, almost everyone around you falls right in with the act, oohing and
ahhing at the naked emperor rather like the courtiers
in the fable.

I was, I think, a particularly laughable figure in
those days. I had assiduously cultivated a no-nonsense, authoritative air, reinforced by a hairdo in
which every lock was pulled back from my face,
straight and severe, and coiled into a precise bun
dead center atop my head. This style was intended to
make me appear older and more imposing, more professional. It was a look I thought befitting a woman
doctor. I affected a brisk, efficient manner and spoke
in clipped tones. I was a terribly important, terribly
busy, terribly competent person. My aping of the
stereotype of the passionless, cold-as-ice woman of
science was almost perfect. But there were those
glasses. I had, after much internal debate, traded my
sensible, horn-rimmed glasses in for a pair of those
plastic-framed affairs popular at the time (at least
among certain sets), the kind that had wing tips,
rather like the tailfins on old Cadillacs, swooping
up from the outer edges of the frame on either side.
Highlighting this lovely look was a spray of rhine-
stones embedded in the plastic of the wing tips. I
thought them madly elegant and imagined that they
added a touch of feminine glamour to my image. (I
had, in those days, a great deal of imagination.)

I must have been an amusing figure, clipping
about, briskly efficient, all business, with those ludicrous glasses so completely at odds with my
no-nonsense manner. But no one laughed at my af-
fectations. My patients certainly didn't. Who wanted
to think that the doctor, the person to whom you'd

entrusted your health, the person who you were perhaps going to allow to cut into your very insides, was, after all, rather an ass. No, the patients did not laugh. And the nurses and the rest of the staff had been trained, no matter how it went against the grain, to act as if the doctor were some elevated being, always in the right.

Everyone seemed to have a high opinion of me: The patients whose babies, despite all threatening complications, I managed to deliver safe and whole into their arms; the women who, by a few simple strokes of my scalpel, I managed to rid of their pain; and the infertility patients who, after what was often years of barrenness, I managed to get pregnant. Yes, as curious as it sounds, we really did think of it that way—as if *we* had gotten them pregnant. It's a prevalent fantasy among gynecologists. "Oh, yes " we say, "I got her pregnant." Husbands and lovers recede into the background—or sometimes even participate in the doctor's fantasy out of gratitude. In short, there are so many grateful patients telling us how wonderful we are that it's hard not to agree.

Of course, at bottom we know that what we do is generally not all that miraculous or special. Most of it is actually quite routine and ordinary; a farm wife disemboweling, quartering and boning a chicken or a butcher preparing a cow for market possesses essentially the same skills. But the whole business of medicine is surrounded by such a mystique, shrouded in so many obscure polysyllabic Latin terms, that it usually seems to the uninitiated to be much more than it is, and the doctor, likewise, comes off as a mysterious, all-knowing, quasireligious figure, an illusion aided by our white coats, our medical mumbo jumbo, our exaggerated air of authority. In our heart of hearts, we may know that we're merely acting out an elaborate charade, but, amid all that uncritical admiration, it's easy to begin to lose touch with reality, to become somewhat less than humble. Yes, of course it's all a sham, but it's so seductive, all that approval and admiration, that you find yourself suddenly all puffed up with your own hot air. You begin, in short, to believe your own PR.

They say there is a god who watches over fools and drunkards, and my own experience confirms this, for *somebody* certainly was looking out for the particular sort of fool I was becoming—so dangerously full of my self that I was about to lose all sense of gravity and float right off the face of reality. And, with a sharp kindness, this god loosed a barb keen enough to prick and deflate my overblown ego. Or maybe not—but it's hard to believe that Mrs. Sampson's coming into my life at that time wasn't destined.

Just when I was beginning to fancy myself the great white hope of gynecology, Mrs. Sampson called the GYN clinic and made an appointment, saying specifically that she wanted an appointment with me. Mrs. Sampson was the wife of one of the biggest of the bigwigs in my little world, a man at the top of the hospital administration. If she'd needed a hangnail removed, she could have requested and gotten the chief of surgery to do the operation. Her high position meant she had access to insiders' information, and the fact that she'd undoubtedly tapped that ultimate source of information and had as a consequence requested an appointment with me was the highest form of flattery.

Mrs. Sampson looked like an advertisement for something sleek and expensive, and, given my current investment in the prerogatives of hospital hierarchy and status, I expected someone rather queenly and imperious. But she was in fact a charming, warm, unassuming woman. Her case was not really an unusual one, except that she was rather young to be having this particular problem—a prolapsed uterus, a condition in which the uterus prolapses, or falls out of its normal position. Mrs. Sampson's prolapse was so severe that her uterus had fallen well into the vaginal cavity. It was obvious to me that she was going to need a hysterectomy.

She had three children and didn't want any more, so the prospect of losing her uterus at the age of thirty-five was not as upsetting as it might have been. I recommended a vaginal hysterectomy, which was the usual procedure in such cases, but even in cases as obvious as Mrs. Sampson's, we had to get a second opinion. Third-year residents sent anyone they saw whom they felt needed surgery to the chief for the second opinion. I arranged a consultation with him.

Normally, assuming the chief concurred with me about the need for surgery, the case would be passed back to me, and, because I was now a senior resident, I would perform the operation, assisted by one of the other senior residents rather than by the chief or a staff doctor. Every once in a while, though, a patient would balk at being referred back to a female surgeon. It was all fine and good to have a woman doctor prescribe some birth control pills or do your yearly checkup, but when it was something serious, something requiring surgery . . . well, then you wanted someone *really* competent, and in those preliberated days a fair number of women just couldn't accept the notion that a woman surgeon could be as competent as a man. The chief always stuck up for me and tried hard to convince the doubters to allow me to do their surgery. Usually, they would give in to the chief, but occasionally a woman would be really adamant about not having a woman surgeon, and I would lose the case.

The chief always told me when a woman I'd referred to him expressed anxiety at the idea of having another woman operate on her. But he'd take the sting out of it by telling me, "She didn't like the idea, Jane"—and this obviously amused him—"but I told her you were the best surgeon I had and she came around.''

I didn't get the feeling from Mrs. Sampson that she'd be hesitant about having a woman surgeon. But, because Mrs. Sampson was such a VIP, I assumed that the chief would do the operation himself, with one of the staff doctors assisting him. Even though I understood and accepted the politics of the situation, I was disappointed, because I'd been on the surgery ward for almost a month now and Mrs. Sampson was the first vaginal hysterectomy to come my way. I'd done several abdominal hysterectomies in the past month, but no vaginals. I don't know exactly why I was so eager to do a vaginal hysterectomy. I'd done plenty of vaginals as a second-year resident and was quite proficient at the procedure. The only difference would be that another senior resident, rather than the chief or a staff doctor, would assist on any vaginals I now did—which was really no difference at all. But with an adolescent eagerness, I was looking forward to doing my first vaginal as a chief resident. I was like a young girl yearning after her first pair of high heels. Somehow it was going to make me more grown-up, not just a kid doctor anymore. It was a completely ridiculous attitude, but oh, I had itchy fingers. I went about cursing my bad luck to anyone who would listen, which was practically nobody.

I was still sulking a couple of days later when the chief told me to fit Mrs. Sampson into my OR schedule.

''I offered to do it myself, of course. She wouldn't hear of anyone else but you operating on her. Amazingly tactful woman, though—I'm only half as insulted as I should be. What with you youngsters breathing down my neck, I'll be put out to pasture before I know it.'' The chief pretended to grumble; and maybe he *was* a bit miffed. I noticed he didn't offer to assist on the operation, but I think his miff, if any, was mingled with pride in this hotshot young woman doctor that he himself had recruited and trained.

At any rate, I did the operation—brilliantly, if I do say so myself. And say it I did. Not that I ran around buttonholing people and telling them, nothing so crass. But I did manage to find a couple of opportunities to mention casually that the operation had taken only half an hour. Doing a "vag hyst" in only a half an hour was a snazzy piece of business. It was becoming quite clear to me that I really was something rather special: a cut above, as it were. I took to admiring my hands and patting myself on the back. There was a more pronounced swing to my swagger.

On her fourth day post-op, Mrs. Sampson developed a slight fever. I wasn't terribly concerned. A slight infection as a complication in a vag hyst is not unusual. You're making an incision in the vagina in order to get into the sterile pelvic cavity to get at the uterus, and there is no way to completely sterilize the vagina. Such post-op infections are especially common in premenopausal women who still have a good blood supply to that area. Some of the germs from the vagina get up in there, and blood being the perfect breeding ground, an infection develops. I ordered antibiotics. On the fifth day Mrs. Sampson continued running a fever, and it was half a degree higher. I ordered more antibiotics. On the sixth day, Mrs. Sampson's fever was spiking. When the fever goes down a bit each day, you know you're doing just fine, and if it only holds steady, still you're not losing ground. But when it starts spiking up and up, you're in trouble.

I began pouring every antibiotic known to medical science into Mrs. Sampson's veins. I couldn't figure out what was happening. I kept examining her, feeling for a hot spot that would localize the infection for me, but I couldn't find anything. Usually the infection is at the top of the vagina, right where you've made the incision, and you'll get some pus to drain out. But Mrs. Sampson's incision felt and looked just fine.

Meanwhile, Mrs. Sampson was not at all fine. I was poking around in that infected tissue, stirring things up, and her fever was climbing. She was also getting sicker in reaction to all the antibiotics I was pumping into her. Her pulse was rapid, her blood pressure was out of whack.

The chief had been out all week with a bad flu, and when I finally called him at home, I could hardly make out what he was saying.

"It sounds to me like you've got a patient with an ovarian abscess, Jane," he croaked.

Terrific, an ovarian abscess. Mrs. Sampson's ovary was infected, and there was a big abscess full of pus sitting in her ovary. No antibiotic in the world was going to touch it, because the blood supply to the ovary just isn't sufficient to allow the antibiotic to get into the abscess and fight the infection. So, I had to take Mrs. Sampson back into the operating room and remove the infected ovary.

"Do whatever you need to do to make me better, Doctor," she said. Mrs. Sampson still thought I was the great doc.

Mrs. Sampson was fine after the operation to remove her ovary, but I wasn't doing too well. My overgrown ego came tumbling down on top of me, nearly crushing me with its excessive weight. I suppose if I hadn't been so unrealistically puffed up in the first place, I might not have been so deflated by what were, after all, quite common complications. An *E. coli* infection of the ovary can happen even to the best of surgeons. In performing the hysterectomy I'd gotten in and out of there with admirable speed, thus doing a lot towards reducing the chances of infection. But despite my speed, some *E. coli*, a normal inhabitant of the vagina, had gotten up there and infected the ovary. I knew it could have happened to anyone;

but I also knew that good surgeons, really skilled ones, have a rate of infection lower than the norm. They traumatize less tissue, and therefore have a lower rate of infection. I was sure that something in the way I'd handled that ovary was responsible for the fact that it had gotten infected.

I didn't think it was possible to feel any more miserable than I was feeling in the week or so after Mrs. Sampson's discharge. God's Gift to Gynecology done in by miserable microscopic bacteria! I was on a steady diet of humble pie, a dish that had been missing from my menu for some time.

As it turned out, it was possible to feel more miserable. About a week after Mrs. Sampson's discharge, I saw another patient with severe prolapse. The chief agreed she was a candidate for a vaginal hysterectomy. I did the operation, and this woman also developed an *E. coli* infection. This time the infection was at the incision in the vagina and wasn't so severe. She quickly got better—and I got worse.

The chief started making jokes about Typhoid Mary and took to calling me *E. coli* Jane. I think he meant by his joke to show me that he had confidence in me. Certainly he wouldn't have considered it a laughing matter if he thought that something in my technique had caused these infections. His jokes did not, however, cheer me up. My confidence had hit low ebb. I wasn't sure I could walk and chew gum at the same time, let alone do surgery.

EIGHT

M Y LACK-OF-CONFIDENCE attack was severe, but
not terminal. Enough vaginal hysterectomies
came and went sans *E. coli* so that I eventually
recovered. And, of course, it was in the end a very
good thing, having the wind taken out of my sails like
that. It saved me from a fate I've seen other surgeons
fall prey to: when their comeuppance arrived, as it inevitably does, their firmly entrenched sense of their
own infallibility leaves them blaming all complications arising from their surgeries on someone else—a
nurse, a lowly intern, the patient herself.

At any rate, by the time I'd recovered, it was the
middle of my third and final year of residency, and I
was faced with a major career decision. In six months
my training would be over; I'd have to decide what I
was going to do with myself.

It rained a good deal that winter as it does some
years, pouring out of the sky in great hard bucketfuls.
It was a deluge of unmanageable proportions for a
city that is really nothing more than an irrigated strip
of desert at the edge of a great sea. It washed the mud
off the hillsides, flooded the canyons, carried away
homes and even left cars perched in treetops; it cre-
ated tremendous chaos. And my life was in perfect
harmony with the weather that winter.

Trying to decide what to do, as if there were a great
many options to choose from—and theoretically there
were—I spent hour after hour watching raindrops

splat against the windows and run down the panes in sheets.

I could choose to go into private practice, hanging up my shingle in some likely area, one not already overrun with gynecologists. But I had no money to rent and furnish an office, no rich parents to stake me; and even with bank loans, I would have needed some sort of cash to tide me over until my practice was established. But more than that, there was the fear that I would sit there in my office for a year or two waiting for the phone to ring and patients to come in. Maybe the patients would never show; my being a woman gynecologist was then not an asset. And, the business side of running a private practice intimidated me. In those days, it was common knowledge that women had no head for business. They could barely balance their checkbooks, poor things. I would hear over and over again tales of women doctors fallen into financial disarray because of their inability to develop a head for business. (I have often wondered what a head for business must look like: I envision a cash box mouth and register eyes.) Running my own practice sounded seductive, but the attraction was not sufficient to overcome my fear of such independence. So private practice was not really an option.

There was also the option of getting a salaried staff position as an attending physician at some government or university hospital, but that would have been the same as being an intern—patients constantly in and out, usually only seen on an emergency basis, then gone forever; no real continuity. Perhaps the most appealing option was that of joining an already established private practice as a junior partner. This was the option that most of the residents chose. The business details would vary, but generally, an established doctor, his practice bursting at the seams, would invite a young doctor just out of residency to work for him at a certain salary, and perhaps a percentage of the business as well, for a year or two, the idea being that the percentage would grow each year until the young doctor became a full partner. Unfortunately, doctors weren't beating down my door begging me to join their practice. In fact, I didn't have a single inquiry, because, as already noted, women gynecologists were not of great value on the open market at the time.

The last option was to stay on where I was, joining the medical plan staff at the hospital. The advantages were manifold. The salary was generous. I wouldn't have to invest any money in setting up a practice. I would be assured of plenty of patients. There'd be no tangling with accountants and billing and quarterly tax forms. Moreover, I would be able to practice medicine without any thought of expense to my patients. If I needed a lab test or an X ray or whatever, it would be covered by the monthly fee paid by patients and their employers. Besides, I'd been there for three years. I liked it. It was comfortable and safe. It was, I decided, altogether the best thing.

This option had only one major flaw—no one had offered me the job. The chief, who was head of the staff and would have been the one to extend an offer of employment, hadn't given the slightest indication that he'd like me to stay on. He hadn't offered so much as a casual "What are your plans for the future?"—which is why I spent so much time staring at raindrops that winter.

Initially I told myself that it was merely a matter of time, that soon he would call me in and make me an offer of a staff position. But the weeks wore on, and he didn't. I thought fleetingly of taking the situation in hand and asking instead of waiting for the chief to make the first move, but that would have been impossible for me. It was more than just the fear of rejection, although that in itself was powerful enough to have deterred me: After all, what would I have done

if I'd asked for a staff position and been refused?
Quite clearly, the world would have ended. But, before even that fear, there was the simple impossibil-
ity, the impropriety, of my going to the chief and
asking for a job. It would have been . . . well . . .
somehow unladylike, an act of assertion beyond my
ken. So I waited demurely and in vain for an invitation. But for one of the nurses, I might have gone demurely on to some dreary staff position at a backwater
hospital, working night and weekend shifts for doctors with prosperous private practices.

It was one of my Friday nights out with the girls.
We were sitting around swizzling the chunks of fruit
about in our exotic canned pineapple juice tropical
drinks, and during a lull in the conversation one of
the nurses, Susan Pratt, asked me what my plans
were for the next year. Everyone at the table turned to
look at me, and maybe it was the rum in the drinks,
but most uncharacteristically I found myself blurting
out that no one wanted me in private practice, and I
didn't think I could make a go of it on my own, and
I'd been scouring the ads in the back pages of the
medical journals, but everyone knows those ads were
dreary, dead-end, last-resort jobs, and what I really
wanted to do was stay on at the hospital, but the chief
hadn't said beans to me about it—all this in practically
one breath.

"But Jane, don't you know?" Susan asked, still
laughing as she spoke.

"Know what?" I said, sulky and stung by the
laughter.

"About the chief's policy. He never asks any of the
residents to stay on."

"He thinks it wouldn't be fair," Ginny, another of
the nurses, explained, "putting undue pressure on
the residents and that sort of thing. Afraid the residents might stay on out of allegiance to him, rather

than making the best career decision for themselves. You know how he is.''

The next morning, I went in to see the chief and told him I wanted to stay on. He beamed at me. I beamed back at him. Of course, there was the formality of the staff having to vote me into the partnership, but he could practically assure me a job.

It was not the first time a nurse had influenced the course of my career, and it wouldn't be the last.

So, on July first, 1968, I officially joined the staff at the hospital. I went through my usual quaking in my boots number at the idea of my enlarged responsibilities, but actually my life didn't change much. I wasn't working quite as many hours. I was only on call once every two weeks, but I still had to be at the hospital from early in the morning till five or six at night. There were still evening meetings and Saturday mornings.

Now, however, I was making a good deal more money—but somehow that fact hadn't quite registered. I still lived in the same dreary, rat infested neighborhood, in the same boxy apartment with the same grey rented furniture. The only difference was that when I balanced my checkbook each month there were all these extra digits. Instead of having ten bucks to last till next payday, there were these hundreds, and then thousands of dollars in my checking account. I'd been wearing surgical scrub suits for eight years, so I went out and bought some clothes, but you can buy only so many clothes, and the balance in my checking account just kept getting bigger and bigger. I was having to write smaller and smaller just to fit the balance into the tiny space in my check recorder. I had no idea what to do with money. Money simply wasn't very real to me. I think, too, I had the same block a lot of women have about money. Money, like it or not, has some sort of equation with power in our culture, and at that point in my life, it was not a sort of power I could own.

I had been living a student's hand-to-mouth existence for twelve years, and although a medical student's, intern's or resident's salary is practically poverty level, it's not a grinding, soul-depressing poverty; you know it's just temporary. So I just went on living my studentesque life-style, letting what seemed to me like vast sums of money reside in my checking account.

I had completed four years of college, four years of medical school, a year's internship, a three-year residency. My period of training was officially over, but in my mind I wasn't finished, and I still thought of myself as a student. There was one last hurdle, one more thing I had to accomplish, before I would be truly finished in my own mind, and that was board certification.

Board certification is a special honor. Each of the various medical specialities has a board that certifies doctors in its field. A doctor who has graduated from a board-approved medical school, served a board-approved internship and completed a board-approved residency program can apply to take the board certification qualifying exams.

For Obstetrics and Gynecology, the exams are in two parts. The first part is a written examination, which you can take as soon as you finish your residency. The second part is an oral examination, and if you've passed the written exam, you can take the orals, but not until you've been in practice for two years following the completion of your residency. You then submit to the board a record of all the cases requiring hospitalization that you've treated during those first two years. Provided your record is clean— you haven't done something so heinous as mangling or killing a patient—you then get to take the oral part of the exam, which is administered by the country's top-notch gynecologists.

Being board certified means that you are one of the elite, the crème de la crème of your speciality. Board certification is not mandatory. It's not like the exams you *have* to take to be licensed to practice medicine; it's voluntary. Not everyone tries for it, and of those that do, only about half make it. But it wasn't really voluntary for me. It was something I *had* to do. For me, board certification was going to be the culmination of my medical career. It was going to be the final visible proof to everyone, myself included, that even though I was a woman, I was good. All the secret doubts and terrors that swam like luminous monsters beneath my surface satisfactions would be securely locked away forever if only I could nail down this one last official certificate announcing that Dr. Jane Patterson was certified by the Board of Obstetricians and Gynecologists. That thin piece of parchment, embossed and beribboned, neatly framed and hung on my office wall, was going to exorcise the demons of self-doubt once and for all. I had a lot riding on the qualifying exams.

At the earliest opportunity I applied to take the written exam, and studied for months. As the time drew near, I took to getting up in the cold milky light of dawn to put in an hour of studying before I had to be at the hospital. I ate lunch riffling through my stack of index card notes. I went home at night and studied some more, falling asleep under the weight of ponderous texts.

I got compulsive about it, covering the walls of my apartment with thumbtacked notes. I had everything systematized. My kitchen was the ovary. The refrigerator was covered with operative diagrams depicting a hundred and one surgical techniques for slicing away at the ovary. The wall above the stove was ovarian tumors, both cancerous and noncancerous. Infections of the ovary were pinned above the dish drainer. Hermaphrodites and other bizarre chromosomal abnormalities festooned the breakfast alcove. The north wall of the living room was the vulva; the south wall the uterus and fallopian tubes. The east and west were taken up by the vagina and the cervix, respectively. Obstetrics took up the entire bedroom. Menstrual disorders and sexually transmitted diseases hung in the bathroom. Infertility was in the narrow, dark entry that led from the front door to the living room. "Benign and Malignant Ovarian Tumors," hanging over the stove, caught fire one day and brought the landlady pounding at the door. It was nothing, really nothing at all, I tried to explain, just some ovaries I'd overcooked.

I passed the written exams, and for a while, I cooled off, but as the orals drew closer, the same maniacal compulsiveness took over. I fretted over the hospital case records I'd submitted to the board. Should I have operated sooner on this case? Why had that woman been readmitted to the hospital for a postoperative complication? How would I explain these things? I began having the kind of anxiety dreams college students have—the ones in which it's the end of the semester and you've just discovered that you signed up for a course, but somehow forgot all about it and never went to the class, and now you are going to flunk. I even went back to my favorite grade school anxiety dream, of going to school and all of a sudden realizing I'd forgotten to get dressed and had come to school stark naked.

I buttonholed everyone I knew who'd been through the exams. What advice did they have? They all had different advice. "Don't worry about that area," one would tell me, "concentrate on this." So I would, and the next person would say, "No, forget about this, concentrate on that." I became pathologically suggestible. The only truly useful advice I got was from one of the staff doctors who had once been an examiner for the oral boards.

"Two things, Jane," he told me, "only two things you have to remember. One—if you don't know something, say so, because if you don't know, they're going to find out, so don't try and stonewall it. Admit you don't know, cut your losses, and go on to the next question.

"Two—don't argue with the examiner. If he's asked you how to prevent ovarian cancer and you've given an answer and he says, 'Oh, no, the best way to prevent ovarian cancer is to remove everyone's ovaries at birth,' don't argue. Just say that although it's not an approach you're familiar with, now that you think about it, it sounds like a swell idea."

The board qualifying exams were held in Chicago. I arrived the day before, so I'd be able to get a good night's sleep. Hah!

First thing in the morning, all the candidates were herded into the hotel's conference room, where we sat for hours awaiting our turn. Everyone else was as nervous and dry-mouthed as I. There were long lines at the drinking fountains and longer ones outside the bathrooms. It was one of those rare moments in my career when being a woman was actually an advantage. I didn't have to wait in line to pee.

Everyone sat in this cavernous room, some silent, some chattering nervously. The conversational murmur would rise to a certain nervous peak, and then a man in a black suit would march to the front of the room and, like the town crier announcing ruin in Pompeii, call out a name in a thunderous baritone that cut through the chatter like a surgical knife. Dead silence would follow as hundreds of eyes turned to watch the condemned rise and leave the room. Then the volume of chatter would begin to build again, until the next name was called.

Finally the words I'd waited for so long to hear—

"Dr. Jane Patterson"—were called, and I followed the man in the black suit out to the elevators and up to the fourth floor.

"In here," he said, gesturing towards the door to a two-room suite. In the first room was one of the two junior examiners. The examiners could ask whatever they wanted, whenever they wanted, but the basic format was that in the first room the questions would be about general gynecological and obstetrical knowledge, and in the second room the questions would center on the hospital records you'd submitted. There was a junior examiner in each of the two rooms and a senior examiner who floated in and out, disconcertingly popping off questions whenever the whim struck.

In the first room there was a screen and a projector and the examiner would show a slide of some diseased organ or a microscopic sliver of tissue, and you'd have to say what the disease was.

"Uh, those are chorionic villi, and they've penetrated beyond the uterine wall, so that must be trophoblastic disease," I said, looking at the first slide.

The examiner made a noncommittal grunt, and on and on we went through ruptured ectopic pregnancies, cervical dysplasia, luekoplakei vulvitis, adenomatous hyperplasia, germinal inclusion cysts, serous cystoadenomas, adenomyosis, lymphogranuloma venereum, ad infinitum, punctuated only by the examiner's grunting sounds, which could have been interpreted to mean either assent or disagreement and sounded rather like the sound a grazing cow might make before moving on to a new patch of grass. Sometimes he would pause at a certain slide.

"Cervical cancer," I offered my diagnosis.

"Describe the spread of cervical cancer through the pelvic lymph nodes."

I began my recital.

"And then, Doctor?" he prompted after I'd delved deep into the chain of pelvic lymph nodes, to the point where my knowledge gave out. I could hear a voice in the back of my head saying, "If you don't know, Jane, say you don't know."

"I don't know, sir," I said.

After what seemed like three lifetimes, he asked me to step into the next room.

The examiner there began by concentrating on cases involving complications, probing my knowledge of the incidence of various complications, the proper steps in the diagnosis and treatment of complications. Next they asked me about a certain case in which I'd operated on a woman who had a growth on her ovary. Any time a woman has an ovarian enlargement there's the possibility of ovarian cancer, and in my preoperative diagnosis, I had written "possible ovarian malignancy." I had done a Pfannenstiel incision, a three- to four-inch incision that runs horizontally across the lower abdomen just above the pubic bone.

"Do you really think, Doctor, that a Pfannenstiel incision allows for adequate visualization of the pelvic cavity?"

Well, of course I thought so; that's why I had done a Pfannenstiel. From the tone of his question though, it was obvious that he was from the school purporting that in order to adequately investigate the pelvic cavity for signs of cancer having spread, you must make a larger, vertical incision from the belly button all the way down to a point just above the pubic bone. I was about to say that I thought the Pfannenstiel was just fine when the voice in the back of my mind reminded me, "Don't argue with the examiner."

"Well," I said, "I was trained to do a Pfannenstiel in such situations, but I'm aware of the literature suggesting that a vertical incision allows for more adequate inspection of the pelvic cavity. Obviously you've had more experience with this than I've had, so I'd have to defer to your superior medical judgment on that.'' My obsequiousness must have struck the right note. He gave me a short lecture on the virtues of the vertical incision and then went on to the next question.

I had an unusual number of hospital admissions, voluminous compared to the number of cases most young doctors have, because I worked as a staff doctor at the medical center of a prepaid health plan. But what really distinguished my hospital case load from that of most other applicants for certification was that, because I'd been practicing in California, I'd done a large number of abortions. At that time, California was one of the few states that had liberalized their abortion laws, and the bulk of the questions the examiners asked me were about abortion procedures and their complications.

And then it was all over. They thanked me and ushered me out of the room, and I made my way out of there on rubber legs.

It was not yet lunchtime. I had a plane reservation to fly that evening to Pittsburgh, where I would spend the weekend with my parents before flying back to LA. But, eager to flee the scene, I grabbed my bags, took a taxi out to O'Hare and caught a noon flight. I buckled my seatbelt and ordered a double martini. I flew through the sky playing mental Ping-Pong with myself: passed, didn't pass, passed, didn't pass. I read volumes into each nuance of the examiners' grunts. They had hated me. I was one of those wicked liberal woman abortionists from crazy California. That's why there'd been so many questions about abortion. It took me years to realize that they'd probably asked all those questions about abortions because none of them had ever done more than a handful and they were simply curious about the procedure. It took me four double martinis to stop worrying about it.

I landed in Pittsburgh, no longer the least bit worried about my board exams—or anything else. The stewardess managed to put me and my carry-on luggage together. I couldn't thank her enough. She was a dear and wonderful person. I told her so several times. I poured myself down the ramp and sloshed into the terminal searching the waiting crowds for my parents. It had been six years since I'd seen them. There hadn't been enough money or time for visits home during the lean years of my internship and residency, but finally, their daughter the doctor was coming home. The shy, quiet, studious girl they'd waved goodbye to six long years ago came swerving into the terminal, and spotted them way down there at the end of the long hallway.

"Hi Mom, Hi Dad," I began yelling at the top of my lungs, lurching towards them.

I can still see them standing there, staring wide-eyed at my approach.

"Whatsamatter, don't you know me? It's me, Jane," I said, dropping my bags and pointing at myself with both hands, as if maybe they'd missed noticing me.

I passed out in the car on the way home from the airport, or as my mother euphemistically put it, I fell asleep. At any rate, I woke up the next morning in my own bed. A caravan of camels had passed through my mouth during the night, or I'd been sucking on nickels in my sleep. Sparrows were chirping in the bushes outside my window. Their song was as melodious as the wild cry of a pterodactyl. Someone had done cruel things to the insides of my skull. It was the first and last time I ever had four double martinis in a row, but my hangover served a purpose. Two in fact. First, my mother tiptoed around me as if she were walking on eggshells, and not once did she ask me when I was planning to come home and get married and produce her grandchildren. Second, so acute was my physical misery that I didn't worry about the board exams once during the entire weekend.

But I made up for lost time once I got back to LA, where I spent eight long weeks worrying about them. The decision is made as soon as you leave the room, but it takes two months to be notified of it. I'm not sure if this is a policy of deliberate kindness or deliberate cruelty. Maybe they wait so that you'll have time to rehearse for the possibility of failure and don't commit seppuku on the spot. Or maybe they string it out for the sadistic pleasure of it. More likely, it's just the slow gait of a lumbering bureaucratic beast that accounts for the delay.

At any rate, it finally came, a form letter with two boxes; one checked if you passed, the other if you hadn't. I had! Hallalooya! Hallay!

NINE

LIFE CAN BE such a perverse bastard. There I was,
thirty years old, and after fourteen long, scrabbling
years, I had finally arrived. I had it all, even my
board certification. I had paid my dues. I was supposed to start living happily ever after. It just didn't
seem right that, instead, a thick grey fog of depression rolled into my life and settled about my shoulders, with no signs of lifting.

I tried to tell myself it was a temporary thing. It was
just that the adrenaline that had kept me busy, busy,
busy for so long was gone now that I no longer had
any goals to goad me on. I was having post-board depression the same way other women have postpar-
tum depression. I simply needed a little time to let my
system readjust, and then it was all going to be okay.

I was like one of those trained dogs in the circus that
run around the ring jumping through hoops. I'd been
jumping through hoops for years, so intent on the
hoops that I didn't even notice I was running around
in circles. Now that the hoops were gone, I was no
longer insulated from that reality. I didn't know
which way to jump.

But, any day now the fog of depression was going
to lift, and there'd be some sunshine in my life again.

Months went by without a single ray. I tried to buy
my way out of it. I don't suppose I really thought it
would work, but at least I could suffer in comfort. I
bought a shiny red, outrageously expensive sports

car, paying cash for it. I felt madly glamorous bopping about the sun-drenched streets of LA, cruising the hills and canyons, the dashing young doctor in her flying machine. But the sports car was like a cold remedy; it provided only temporary, symptomatic relief. It didn't cure the underlying problems.

Not long ago, I read Gail Sheehy's book *Passages*, in which she describes a variety of different patterns that men's and women's lives take as they journey through adulthood. My life had always seemed to me to be so different from the lives of other women. I didn't expect to find myself fitting into any of the patterns that Sheehy found in women's lives. And, on the surface, I didn't. In fact, my life at thirty seemed most akin to the life of a successful male business executive she describes. This man, after years of consumingly ambitious striving, has finally made it. He has it all, only to find that life has become curiously flat and dull, and he wakes up one morning wondering what, if anything, it all means. His life feels empty. It seemed an accurate description of my life at thirty. Never mind that I was thirty and a woman, I was having the sort of male mid-life crisis that is the hallmark of so many successful men in their late forties and fifties.

But upon reflection, I now wonder if my life hasn't followed a more typically female pattern after all. One of the female patterns that Sheehy describes is the woman who spends the decade between twenty and thirty finding a mate and establishing a family. She gives herself over to the needs of others, nurturing her children and supporting her husband's ascending career. After about ten years of feathering the nest, nurturing and supporting others, she finds herself desperately needing to find the self that somehow got submerged beneath dirty diapers and endless emotional outlay for her husband, and tries to find her way back to the center of her own life.

I know the women she means. I see them in my office all the time. They are sometimes confused and inarticulate about what they are trying to do with their lives, but I know exactly what they are talking about. In all those years of nurturing and supporting, they have given away too much of themselves. They want some sense of themselves apart from their husbands and children.

I know the feeling: It was exactly how I felt at that stage of my life. On the surface my life seemed very different from the lives of these women, but the underlying emotional dynamic was the same. My career was husband and kids all rolled into one. As so many women do with their families, I had made too much room for my career. I didn't know who I was apart from my career, mainly because I *wasn't* much of anybody apart from it.

I think the thing that really got me was Journal Club. As a resident, I had been required to show up at Journal Club each month and present summaries of the articles from the medical journals I'd been assigned to read that month, but I was a staff member now, and staff members weren't required to attend. Sitting around listening to residents report on some arcane article detailing the latest developments in the clinical management of malignant and benign vulvar lesions was hardly a hot night on the town. Most of the staff didn't bother to come. But I never missed a one. It was practically the highlight of my social calendar.

Journal Club often met at the chief's house, but sometimes one of the staff doctors would host. I remember those evenings spent in the homes of people I barely knew, sitting on the edge of a brocade straight-backed chair, a teacup or perhaps a glass of wine perched on my knee, listening to the dreary recitals of article summaries while all around me residents and staff doctors sprawled carelessly on furniture and floor, drinking beer and laughing with a lazy camaraderie. I would sit there feeling thin and brittle, like a maiden aunt dusted off and dragged out for the family reunion.

Perhaps I did not come off as distant and stiff as I felt, but I did feel distant, and it was not just the distance from the easy good fellowship of the residents and the doctors; I was used to being on the outside of that inner circle. It was coming into these houses that were homes, where even things—the furniture, the knickknacks on the shelves, the paintings on the walls—had the sort of patina that graces things carefully chosen and loved and used with love. Even the material objects exuded a feeling of belonging and connectedness. It would hit me as soon as I walked in the door, a physical tangible force. When kids would come bursting into the living room, interrupting everything and being shushed and sent off to other rooms I would be overwhelmed by the sense that there were other rooms in the houses and lives of these people; that they had lives that went beyond the walls of the hospital.

I would go home to my sterile apartment and my anonymous rented furniture and my bachelorette refrigerator containing a carton of souring milk and a moldy collection of doggie bags left over from restaurant meals I could not finish. I didn't even have a dog. These people had something in their lives that was missing in mine, and it was my sense of this that finally made me go into psychoanalytic therapy.

Getting myself into therapy was about as easy as getting the proverbial camel through the eye of the needle. I was, as they say in the shrink business, heavily resistant to the idea of therapy. Or, in the parlance of southern California, I was blocking.

Part of my resistance was that therapy, in my mind, was connected with hospital psychiatry wards, where there were *really* crazy (as in psychotic) people, who lay curled up in fetal positions, catatonic, or spent their days and nights ranting off demented gospels of which they were the new messiah. Intellectually, I knew there was a difference between hospitalized psychotics and garden variety neurotics like me. But I'd spent enough time in psychiatric wards to know that it can be a fine line. When I'd worked on those wards, I'd too often found myself secretly understanding what those raving lunatics were ranting about, and that worried me: Maybe I was not all that solidly on the safe side of the fine line.

Mostly, though, I knew that my fears about how maybe I was really after all a raving lunatic myself were blown out of proportion. My resistance came more strongly from my fear of telling someone else all my secrets about myself. This was a risky piece of business, because telling all those secrets to someone else meant telling them to myself, too, and I didn't know if I wanted to do that. I knew there were some big, dark secrets down there that should never see the light of day. Better to let sleeping dogs lie. Things could get out of hand. Control, control, we must maintain control.

So, for a long time, I just thought about therapy without doing anything about it. Finally the fog of depression got so thick and seemed so unbearably unending that there didn't seem to be any other choice. I decided that I'd make at least one appointment and try it and see how it went. Maybe it would only take one or two sessions to get myself straightened out.

I could have made an appointment in the psych clinic at the hospital, but I didn't want anyone at the hospital to know I was going into therapy. I had heard a woman therapist give a talk during my internship, and she seemed nice enough, so I made an appointment with her and rehearsed for it during the intervening two weeks. I showed up at her office, and there was this very ordinary, nice, motherly looking, middle-aged woman who did not have deep-set eyes, a penetrating glance or fangs. I wasn't sure I was in the right place. There was an armchair instead of the black leather couch I'd imagined, and she didn't let loose with a single bit of jargon, not once the whole time. I began to feel a lot more comfortable than I'd thought I would.

"Tell me about yourself," she said as she poured us each a cup of coffee. I gave her the little speech I'd rehearsed about how I was a doctor and my speciality was obstetrics and gynecology; that I'd gone to medical school here and done my internship there and had completed my residency and had recently passed my board certification exams. I cluttered up the room with this recital of facts and ended up by saying that although I basically had what I wanted, I'd been kind of . . . well, depressed . . . and I wasn't sure why . . . And there I trailed off, taking a sip of coffee.

She looked down at her own coffee for a minute, frowning into the cup, and then she looked up at me and said, "You know, I have this intuition about you. It may be all off base, but let me try it out. You feel to me like a person who's been carrying a tremendous burden for a long, long time, and it's been very hard, tremendously hard, and you're tired, all tired out, so very tired."

It wasn't so much the words. It was the way she said it, with this kind, sad look on her face, the corners of her mouth pulled down as though by an infinite weariness, her head nodding gently as she spoke. A soft wave of sympathy and empathy flowed from her to me, washing over me, gently rocking me, and it was somehow okay to be all tired out and in need; and I wanted to say, "Yes, that's exactly how it is," but all that came out of me was a hiccuping, moaning sound followed by a flood of tears. I was suddenly sure I was in the right place.

I remember, with crystal clarity, that much of the first session, but I don't remember much else of what was said. Actually, I don't remember in any specific, chronological fashion what was said during any of the subsequent sessions, either. I don't know if it's possible to tell someone about what happens to you in therapy. Never mind boring them to death—how do you go about organizing into some logical, rational fashion something that is neither logical nor rational? Perhaps I should start with the first concrete, observable changes, since concrete, observable change was what I was after.

I went into therapy with a surgeon's attitude. We would find out whatever it was that was causing this depression, and having found it, it would be a simple matter of cutting it out and being rid of it so that I could go merrily about my life. I figured it would take a couple of months on the outside.

It took seven years of individual and group therapy, and rather than being a process of identifying the problem and amputating it, it was more a matter of finding it and owning it. I was, at times, furiously impatient with the whole process. It seemed that all I did was cry. I was paying this woman a hundred bucks an hour to come to her office and blubber for fifty minutes. It was that stupid, useless Lady of the Lake bitch, taking up all my time, crying her eyes out.

So I would cry and cry, and once my gulping sobs subsided enough, I would apologize for crying, or make a few feeble jokes about how my therapist could start using my tears to wash her car or about how much money it must take to keep her clients in Kleenex. Maybe it was here that I first gave the Lady of the Lake her name and image as I tried to tell my therapist about how I felt inside.

My therapist would say, ''Jane, this Lady of the Lake, as you call her, is all the pain you won't allow yourself to feel.'' This much was obvious to me. ''We need to work on that and help you understand why you're so afraid of these feelings." I didn't need to work on that. I knew exactly why. I tried to make her understand that this feeling part of me was just too dangerous to have around in the world where I was trying to stake out my territory. I kept trying to tell her that there were all these people, some of whom were dying, and there were little babies who died, right at the moment of birth. I had to put up some kind of wall between myself and all that or I'd break into little pieces. Everybody knew that. A doctor had a job to do, and I had to maintain careful emotional control or I wouldn't be of any use to my patients or myself. If I allowed myself to feel all that pain, I'd be crying all the time. If I started doing that, everyone would know I was just another one of those women doctors who couldn't take it.

My therapist didn't argue with me; instead she'd say, "Put the pain over here," pointing to a chair across from me, "and talk to it."

"Talk to it?" I said blankly the first time she told me to do this. This was ridiculous. How do you talk to pain? How do you talk to an empty chair? I was not gifted with a great theatrical sense.

"Put the Lady of the Lake in the chair and tell her you want her to go away," she insisted. I felt like a complete idiot talking to an empty chair, but she was the doctor, so I tried to do what she said.

"I want you to go away." I dutifully delivered my line to the empty chair, with all the emotional force of a stilted actor in a badly rehearsed amateur production. But, with some coaching and direction, I began to catch on. Hesitantly at first, and eventually with full force, I'd find myself yelling at the chair as if there were really someone there, someone I was thoroughly annoyed and disgusted with.

"You are nothing but a simple bitch with a bad attitude. Take a walk, get lost. You are of absolutely no assistance to me. Who needs all this whining and sniveling all the time? It is hard enough without you there moaning and groaning. You think that's going to get us anywhere? There are patients to be taken care of. You are getting in the way of proper medical care. How can I be a good surgeon with you pulling at me all the time with your goddamn crying. You have got to get hold of yourself and calm down and shut up."

Oh, I told her good and in no uncertain terms exactly how I felt about her.

Then my therapist would say, "Okay, now sit in the other chair and be the pain." Putting pain in an empty chair and talking to it was hard enough for me, but *being* pain, and talking back, was beyond my ken. I'd get up, though, and switch chairs. Then I'd sit there dumb—without a word to say.

"Look, this is ridiculous," I'd complain. "I don't know what you want me to say."

"I want you to be the Lady of the Lake, and I want you to *tell* her "—she'd point at the chair I just vacated—"tell her how you feel. Say 'I feel hurt and sad and there's a lot of pain here.' "

A meek, tiny little voice would come out of me, parroting back her words: "I feel hurt and sad and there's a lot of pain here."

I had my doubts about this whole thing. But I think they began to diminish when my therapist decided to get into the act and play the Lady of the Lake. I'd sit in one chair, yelling at her, telling her that I didn't want anything to do with her, that she was a danger to me and to my patients with her emotional, mealy-mouthed blubbering.

My therapist's interpretation of the Lady of the Lake was, to say the least, different from mine. This was not a weak and whining Lady.

"You can say all you want and bluster and bully, but I'm real and I'm here. You can call me the most

useless bitch in six counties, but I'm not going anywhere. I've lived this pain and I have a right to it.
You're just going to have to learn to deal with me."

"I can't afford to have you around. I am a doctor. I
cannot allow my medical judgment to be clouded by
your emotionality," I'd say sententiously. "I am responsible for the lives of these people. I can't have
you nagging at me, pulling at me all the time. You're
going to kill someone!" I'd scream.

"That's a crock of shit. Ain't nobody gonna die
'cause I shed a few tears," my therapist, in the guise
of the Lady, would yell right back.

And I'd start laughing, because when I came up
against this full-blown Lady instead of the whining
Lady and my therapist would give her a voice that
was sassy and strong, I began to see how absurd my
fear was. Of course patients weren't going to die if I
cried, nor would the medical profession be brought to
its knees.

I hate to tell you how much time I spent hopping
back and forth between those chairs, but finally, after
months of this, I began to develop a voice for the Lady
that could stand up for her and talk instead of whine
and plead. I began to see that the doctor part of myself had been bullying the more emotional, feeling
part of myself into submission, but I also saw that I
could no longer ignore my face wet with my own
tears. I also saw how terrified I was of my own feelings, how tightly I kept that part of myself locked
away. And I saw that the rationale I had developed
for why I had to do that was so much hot air.

But I still retained the conviction that if I allowed the
Lady any space at all in my psychic life, I would be utterly overwhelmed and would somehow fail as a doctor.

One night during this period of schizoid scrambling
back and forth between my conflicting selves, I was
on call in the emergency room when the admitting

nurse paged me and told me that a young woman who was supposedly three and a half months pregnant had just come into ER bleeding all over the place. It sounded like a miscarriage, but by the time I got down there, the nurse had taken her blood pressure and discovered it to be one eighty over a hundred and ten. Since the woman had no previous history of high blood pressure, there had to be something more than a miscarriage taking place.

The woman was very pale, and her eyes were practically popping out of her head, but she was quite beautiful. Her name was Alexa Kombronovich. She was of Russian extraction and had a luxurious mane of thick, dark hair. I did a pelvic exam on her, and that's when I knew for sure what was happening. Her uterus was way too large, more the size of a five-month pregnancy.

"Am I going to lose the baby, Doctor?" she wanted to know.

"I'm afraid so," I told her. "You're having a miscarriage."

This wasn't strictly true. She wasn't going to lose her baby because there never was a baby in the first place. Alexa Kombronovich had trophoblastic disease, a rare condition—so rare that in all my years of medicine this was the first case I'd seen. Trophoblastic disease, which is also called a "mole" or a "molar pregnancy" or TRD for short, is a condition involving the trophoblast, the specialized layer of cells on the outside of the sac in which the fertilized egg develops.

In normal pregnancies, the embryo attaches itself to uterine wall by means of this trophoblastic tissue. The trophoblast invades the uterine wall and develops projections called chorionic villi, through which the embryo receives blood and nourishment from the mother.

In TRD, the fetus dies early on, or one never develops at all; but even though the fetus has died or is absent altogether, the trophoblast continues to live and, temporarily, to grow. Since the fetal circulatory system is not functioning, the fluid from the chorionic villi that would normally be absorbed by the fetus is not used, and the villi swell until the uterus is filled with a mass of swollen villi that resemble clusters of pale grapes.

She was losing blood rapidly, and it was hardly the time to go into all of this with her. First we had to get her up to OR and replace the blood, remove the rest of the tissue, and stop the bleeding. I explained that she was miscarrying, that there was no hope of saving the pregnancy, and we got her up to OR.

I cried myself to sleep that night, and it wasn't just about the miscarriage. Perhaps I somehow sensed even then that this was only the beginning of Alexa's troubles, or maybe I sensed the change about to take place in me and cried because I was afraid of changing.

I saw her first thing the next morning. She was well enough to want to know what had happened, and I tried to explain in the simplest, gentlest way. I told her that the fetus had died early on or had never really developed, but that placental tissue had continued to grow, creating the illusion that the pregnancy was still growing.

Luckily, she hadn't actually passed any of the villi. A TRD patient who passes these pale, grapelike clumps of tissue and sees them herself often has the feeling that something monstrously deformed has been growing inside her. Somehow the idea that the fetus had died early on, rather than now, at three and a half months, was a comfort to Alexa.

I let that all sink in for a day or two before I told her the rest of it. Even then, I was a firm believer in telling the patient the whole truth and not trying to shield her as some doctors do, but a person can handle only so much at one time.

The rest of it was that she might have cancer. About one in forty cases of TRD are cancerous. She would have to be followed with weekly blood tests for the next several months. If the level of a hormone known as HCG didn't drop, or if it suddenly rose again, we'd know she had a cancerous form of TRD. Alexa's husband was with her when I told her, and they took it pretty well. They had a lot of questions, of course, and it wasn't easy to explain how being pregnant could possibly cause cancer. Most of their questions were what-ifs, all boiling down to the big one: If she had cancer, then what? I explained that cancerous TRD was one of the types of cancer that we'd had a great deal of success with over the past few years and that we could cure most cases. If she did have cancer, she'd have to undergo several months of chemotherapy, which could be rough, but resulted in a ninety percent success rate.

I made a point of seeing her each evening before I went home, and spent a fair amount of time with the couple because they always had a list of questions that had occurred to them since the shock of the last batch of information wore off, allowing them to think more clearly. They were a nice couple, very much in love and very worried.

She was discharged a couple of days later. It was a month or two after that when she called my office one morning.

"Dr. Patterson, this is Alexa Kombronovich," she said in a worried, tight voice that was trying to sound much braver than it was. "I'm very tired out and weak. I just don't seem to have any energy. I can't eat and my skin is this funny yellow color." She paused here for a moment, but before I could say anything, she was crying. "It means I have cancer, doesn't it?"

"Not at all," I said, trying to sound hale and hearty. "It sounds like you have a touch of hepatitis from the blood transfusions," I told her, making it sound like hepatitis was no more serious than a touch of flu. "Don't worry, but I do want you to come in, so I can take a look at you."

She was a most emphatic shade of yellow, and did, indeed, have a roaring case of hepatitis. I admitted her to the hospital to treat the hepatitis. I also ran the weekly HCG test and ordered a set of X rays. The HCG tests came back sky high. She had cancer. Not only that; the X rays showed that the cancer had already spread to her lungs.

I saw Alexa that evening and told her about the hepatitis, but not about the cancer. For one thing, we couldn't treat her for the cancer until we treated the hepatitis, because the hepatitis was affecting her liver. The chemotherapy is also hard on the liver and giving her chemotherapy while she had hepatitis might kill her. Also, I wanted to tell the husband first. I wanted him to have a chance to adjust to the terrible reality, to gather a support group for himself so he in turn could be supportive of Alexa. And, finally, I just didn't know how I was going to stand there and look her in the eye and tell her that on top of everything else, she had cancer.

I caught up with Alexa's husband that evening before he went in to see her. I explained the test results, telling him that his wife had cancer and that it had spread to her lungs. He turned and walked over to the window, and stood looking down at the traffic for a couple of minutes. He came away from the window all stiff, as though something had gone tight and hard at the center of him. I explained that I hadn't yet told Alexa because we couldn't start the chemotherapy until the hepatitis was cleared up anyway, and it seemed best to wait until she was feeling stronger. I also had some other hard news for him. Her situation was especially critical because of the hepatitis. The cancerous form of TRD is highly curable, provided it is treated promptly. But, if we couldn't get the hepati-

tis cleared up in a week or two and start the chemotherapy, her chances of a cure would be considerably
reduced. He wanted to know what "considerably reduced" meant, and I gave him all the facts and figures. I wanted to keep it at that level, being very calm
and matter-of-fact with him. We agreed to speak to
Alexa together the following evening, and I went
down the hall to the nurses' lounge, hid behind the
lockers and cried and cried.

I had a session with my shrink the next afternoon.
I told her about the Kombronoviches, delivering a
succinct summary of the case and its complications,
as if I were an intern and was presenting the case on
rounds. I went on and on in great medical detail, explaining the exact dosages of chemotherapeutic drugs
I planned to administer when and if I cured the hepatitis.

"It must have been very hard for you to tell her
about the cancer," my therapist said, ignoring all the
medical description. I explained that I hadn't actually
told her yet, that so far I'd only told the husband.

"It must have been very painful for you to have to
tell him that," she said with that long, sad look on her
face.

"Well, of course it was painful," I told her. Here
was this poor couple who a week or so ago had been
happily looking forward to the birth of their first child
and now there wasn't a baby, just this mass of horrible grapelike things and this terrible cancer and
maybe she would die and maybe there was nothing
I could do about it. I told her about crying in the
nurses' lounge after talking with the husband, and I
began crying all over again.

"You don't have to keep all that pain locked up inside you, Jane. You keep putting up that brave front,
but you're just putting up walls between you and the
world. Those walls won't make you safe, Jane, they
just make you boxed in and cut off and alone."

I knew what she was saying was true. "I don't know what else to do," I told her.

"You can do what other people do when they're in pain and hurting. You can cry it out. You can allow yourself to feel what you're feeling."

"I did that yesterday and I'm doing it now," I sobbed.

"You can do it right at the time, when you need to do it. You run away and hide from your feelings and cry in secret corners and wonder why you feel so alone, cut off from everyone around. You've got to learn to own your feelings. They're part of you. They will heal you and help you heal others."

I saw the Kombronoviches that evening. They were together, holding each other and talking softly when I came in the room. I felt just the way I had felt all those years before walking into Sheila Hart's room. I wanted to be anyplace else but there. I said my good evenings, how-are-you's, and cleared my throat.

"You remember we spoke before you left the hospital last time about the necessity of following you with these blood tests at regular intervals?"

She nodded, looking at me with enormous frightened eyes.

"Well, I'm afraid I have some bad news. . . ." Her face crumpled up. She pressed her knotted fist against her mouth like she was trying to keep something from coming out. "Oh, God, no, oh no," she kept saying, clutching at her husband's arm, pulling him towards her as if to shield herself from a blow.

I started talking, too loud and too fast, telling her that it was going to be okay, the chemotherapy would work. The success rate was high, very high—ninety percent. I went babbling on and on. It was all stuff I'd told them before, but I couldn't shut myself up. I kept spewing up this avalanche of facts and figures and cure rate and hopeful reassurance. I needed to fill up every inch of space in that room so there wouldn't be room for anything else.

At one level, I knew I didn't need to be doing all that, that I could hold and touch and cry with these people and that we'd all feel far better for it, but I was still terrified of doing that. It was as though my life depended on keeping the feeling part of me shut down. I didn't know why, but that was how I felt. Once again, I ran away.

TEN

I HAVE an awesome capacity for avoidance. If it hadn't been for therapy, I think I could have gone on running away from myself forever. I hate to think of the isolated, dried up prune I might have become. But I was in therapy, and therapy kept making it harder for me to persist in my old ways.

I saw Alexa Kombronovich twice a day. Her hepatitis finally cleared up, and she started chemotherapy. She was pretty sick after the first round of injections, but was doing as well as could be expected. She was finally able to go home, but each month she was readmitted to the hospital for a few days for another round of chemotherapy.

A lot of my time in therapy was spent talking about how I related to patients. My therapist probed and poked about relentlessly. "Do you ever touch your patients when you give them a difficult diagnosis, Jane, hold their hand or something?"

"No."

"Do you ever touch your patients at all, Jane, other than when you're examining them."

"No."

"Why not?"

"Why not?"

My old answers to that question—all that business about needing to be unemotional and properly distant and professional—didn't seem to work anymore. The Lady of the Lake, nurtured in the safety of therapy sessions, had become too strong to be bullied by my rational, scientific doctor self. She stood right up to all that business, and rather than pleading and whining and begging to be heard, she began to insist. She insisted that emotion and caring were too much a part of me and too much a part of being a good doctor to be ignored. The Lady was making it difficult for me to maintain the ''proper'' professional distance from Alexa Kombronovich. She was one of the first patients with whom I'd had such prolonged, frequent contact, and it was getting harder and harder to see her as just a patient. I saw her almost daily now, four months after her first admission; she was becoming an all too real person to me.

I came into her room one morning. She had just begun her third round of chemotherapy and was sitting up in her bed staring in horror at what she held in her hands. There, in great chunks in her hands and all over her pillow, was her lovely, thick hair. The chemotherapeutic drugs we were giving her were killing the cancer cells in her body, but they were also killing normal, healthy cells, and her hair was falling out. We had discussed this side effect, but discussing it and having it happen are two different things.

''I . . . I . . . I . . .'' she began, and then just moved her mouth wordlessly. This woman had been through so much: the miscarriage, the hepatitis, the cancer, violent nausea from the chemotherapy, the possibility of her own death. There was a terrible, desolate look in her eyes, and shaking her head, she held out her hands, full of her own hair, towards me. This was somehow the final straw for her, the last indignity she was capable of bearing. She seemed to be slipping away to some place I wasn't sure she could come back from. I was afraid for her.

Gently, I took the hair from her hands and laid it on the nightstand. I took her hands in mine and sat on the bed next to her.

"Go on, go ahead and cry," I urged her. She just stared at me as though she didn't know who I was.

"Go on, cry. It's okay. I'm here, Alexa, go on and cry," I said, starting to cry myself. She sat there, lost and bewildered in a world that had become too incomprehensibly horrible for her.

"Cry, Alexa, cry, please cry," I cried, and suddenly she seemed to hear me. She tightened her hold on my hands until her knuckles turned white, and finally great waves of sobs broke from her and she cried and cried and cried.

The crying was therapeutic for her and for me. Alexa Kombronovich went through seven months of chemotherapy. It was dreadful. She lost all her hair. She developed huge open sores on her mouth, so that at times we had to feed her intravenously.

But she lived. The cancer was finally gone from her body, and a few years later she gave birth to a lovely, healthy son. The experience of crying with her was like the final untying of a great knot inside me. The medical profession was not brought to its knees. I did not turn into a horrible doctor. My fears were finally laid to rest, and I no longer hesitated to touch my patients, and hold them and cry with them.

I don't think I would have been able to untie this knot if I had not at the same time also been untying some other knots inside me. I had finally gotten to the point in my therapy where I was ready to deal with the biggie: sexuality. Sexuality was not something I could talk about with any ease—a thunderous understatement. To give you an idea: At the end of my first year of residency, the chief had sent Tom Braxton, another first-year resident, and me to the annual conference of the American College of Obstetricians and Gynecologists as a reward for having doubled up on shifts for a time when two of the first-year residents had to leave the program. Tom and I were to attend as many of the workshops and lectures as possible, and when we got back, we would share what we'd learned with the rest of the staff at one of the Thursday afternoon educational meetings. Tom and I divided up and covered as much as possible, but we both attended the keynote address. The keynote speakers at the conference that year were Masters and Johnson. Nobody knew exactly what they were going to say, but everyone knew it would have to do with S-E-X. They spoke to a standing room only crowd.

When we got back to the hospital, Tom and I took turns at the podium presenting what we'd learned. It fell to me to summarize the Masters and Johnson talk. I got up and started to speak, but I just could not stand before a roomful of men and talk about sex. I got to the point where I had to say the word *orgasm*, and my mouth kept moving, but no sound came out. Tom must have understood, for he stepped in saying something entirely gracious like, "Jane, I see you don't have your notes. I have mine right here. Why don't you let me summarize the Masters and Johnson." I could have hugged him.

I suppose most women who grew up in my era have some difficulty in dealing with sexuality. It was an era still essentially Victorian, when women were not supposed to touch, look at, think about or even know their genital organs existed. Sex was still a dark and guilty mystery; in general it was dirty, bad and wrong. .

But my sexuality in particular was problematic. Though I wasn't entirely willing to acknowledge it even to myself, I knew I was a lesbian, and that knowledge was a great tight knot inside me.

I think it first began to dawn on me during adolescence that I was maybe a little bit different from the rest of the girls. My girlfriends were all gaga about this boy or that, but I found myself dazzled not by the star quarterback, but by the head cheerleader. I had never heard the word *lesbian* and had no idea there was such a thing, but I knew girls were supposed to like boys, not other girls. I knew enough to keep my fantasies to myself.

I thought I was the only one in the world. Teenage sexuality is such a bumbling, fumbling, embarrassing thing even for heterosexuals; for gay people it is terrible. I look back now and ache for the lonely little girl I was.

I remember finally discovering there was a word for what I was. I was a voracious reader in my adolescence, and somehow or other I came across a book called *The Well of Loneliness*. Every single lesbian I've ever known has read *The Well of Loneliness*. I don't know how we all manage to find it, but we all do. I read it in bed under my covers with a flashlight way into the night. It is a perfectly horrible book, full of the worst and most damaging stereotypes. The heroine is a woman named Stephen. Her father, wanting a boy, has given her a boy's name and raised her as a boy. She has a severe gender identification problem, which is not what lesbianism is about at all. Anyhow, she is sexually attracted to women, and all sorts of awful things happen to her and the whole thing ends up in some tragic mess, the details of which now escape me. But it didn't seem to matter then that the book was so guilty and sick; the important thing was that *I wasn't the only one*. There was a name for what I was, and, yes, it was dirty and perverted and shameful and wrong, but I was not a lone freak. There were other perverts in the world!

My brother, Fred, had completed medical school and his internship and had begun the first year of his residency in psychiatry. He was living at home at that time, and I would sneak into his room and snitch his textbooks, leafing desperately through indexes looking for the word *lesbianism*. By the time I graduated from high school, I was thoroughly steeped in the psychiatric school of thought on the topic. Lesbianism was a disease, and it arose from an arrested sexual development. Many girls go through a stage of being sexually fixated on other girls. This was quite natural and acceptable. As they matured, their sexuality matured, and their sexual feelings were directed towards the opposite sex. Lesbians, for a variety of reasons, depending on your choice of analytic schools, were arrested in their sexual development, and *this* was neither natural nor acceptable.

I went to bed at night and prayed to God to unarrest me. "Please, God, please, make me not a lesbian." God wasn't listening. I tried to comfort myself with the notion that I was merely a late bloomer, and any day now I was magically going to mature and find my romantic fantasies turning to men. I did not mature.

I had my first affair with another woman in college. I still marvel that lesbians ever manage to find each other, admit to each other that they are gay and actually form romantic, passionate attachments. I can still remember the riskiness of it. We sat in the college cafeteria, and she asked me if I had heard about two seniors who, according to the dormitory scuttlebutt, were lovers. I hadn't, and said so.

Well, what did I think about it? she wanted to know. I gave a learned discourse, gleaned from Fred's textbooks, on the arrested sexual development of lesbians, and said it was probably just a phase they were going through, and it wasn't such a terrible thing to be going through a phase, was it? And then we looked into each other's eyes and allowed ourselves a phase with each other.

Somehow or other Fred caught on, and one weekend when he and I were home alone—my parents had gone somewhere—he said in a dreadfully portentous tone, "Jane, I want to talk to you about something." I had mostly outgrown my puppy dog–like devotion to Fred, but he was still a terribly important and trusted figure. He *accused* me of being a lesbian, and I *con-*

fessed—a very bad move on my part. He threatened to tell our parents. "Oh, no, not that—oh no, *anything* but that," I begged like the heroine in a bad melodrama. Fred relented. If I would stop this monstrous perversion, he would keep quiet. But if I persisted, he would be forced to tell not only my parents, but also the dean of the medical school to which I'd recently been accepted. Oh, I would change! I would drop it like a bad habit. Really I would.

I sneaked around like a criminal for months. My lover and I developed code words to fool Fred, who listened in on my phone conversations. I had a girlfriend who was willing to cover for me. I could pretend to go over to her house, and clandestinely meet my lover. She had no idea I was gay; she thought I was having a love affair with a married man. I didn't disabuse her of that notion.

Fred was from the all-she-needs-is-a-good-lay school of thought on lesbians, and arranged any number of dates for me. I wasn't willing to give up my lover, but I *was* willing to play the game. In the early sixties, the prevailing sexual ethic held that nice girls didn't do it. My sexual willingness must have come as a distinct shock to my sex-starved dates who were accustomed to going to great lengths to get a girl to "go all the way." Here was a girl who would "put out" at the first overture. I was quite popular.

It wasn't that I didn't like sex with men. Contrary to the psychiatric literature on lesbians, I wasn't frigid with men. And I had orgasms. Nowadays, thanks to Masters and Johnson and Shere Hite, we all know that the old reliable in-and-out missionary position doesn't provide enough clitoral stimulation for the vast majority of women to achieve orgasm; only about ten percent of women actually experience orgasm this way. I was even among that ten percent who had these "look ma, no hands" orgasms; but sex with men just wasn't the same as sex with women.

Still, I was encouraged by my first heterosexual experiences. I wasn't frigid, so maybe, after all, I *would* outgrow my homosexual perversions and turn into a normal, natural heterosexual. At that point, I still longed to be heterosexual.

It was through Fred's ministrations that I met my fiancé, John. I enjoyed sex with him. He kept Fred off my back, too, and provided me with a cover and a badge of normality. Meanwhile I carried on a secret love affair. When John asked me to marry him, I said yes. My lesbian lover was also engaged to be married. I really did think it might be possible for me to get married and become a normal heterosexual female; I *wanted* to think it was possible. Then, my lover actually did get married, and I was devastated at losing her.

Reluctantly I made plans for my own marriage. Actually, I didn't have to make plans; my fiancé took care of all that, right down to planning the menu for the wedding reception. John was also planning my career: I would apply for an internship at the university where he worked, and he would see to it that I was accepted. I could specialize in pediatrics, a speciality appropriate for women. It was not as demanding as some specialities, John said; lots of women doctors went into pediatrics. It would allow me to work part-time while I was raising our children. We would have two children, the first one after I'd completed my residency, the second two years later.

I went away that summer to work for a pharmaceutical company in Michigan. All summer long I received letters from my fiancé mapping out the details of my future. I wasn't entirely without a say in these plans. He did ask me whether I wanted slivered almonds in the French-style string beans to be served at the reception. I really couldn't make up my mind about the slivered almonds. I spent the summer thinking about the almonds, and ultimately realized that it wasn't actually the almonds I couldn't decide about. I broke my engagement when I came back to medical school that fall.

I had another brief affair with a woman, and even though it ended, I now knew I wasn't going to turn into a heterosexual. I think the main reason that I decided to apply for an internship three thousand miles away from home was that I knew that I had to get away from my parents and Fred and my hometown if I was ever going to be free to be who I was.

So I moved to California, but the internship was so demanding that I didn't have time for any romantic involvements, heterosexual or homosexual. And, as fate would have it, my brother also wound up in California. Fred finished his residency in psychiatry and was fulfilling his military service obligation by working in a psychiatric clinic at a naval base.

I didn't see much of Fred. There was, to say the least, a certain strain on our relationship. But Fred once again took it upon himself to monitor my sexuality. At the time I was celibate, but I did have women friends and acquaintances. Fred was sure that I was having mad, passionate affairs with them all. In long and tearful scenes, Fred demanded that I confess and repent, and I swore I was on the straight and narrow.

Fred died a few years later of alcoholism, and now, after all these years, I can feel compassion for him. Before he died, he took to bringing men home from the bars where he was quietly and desperately drinking himself to death. Supposedly these "buddies" of his would sleep on the couch. I realize now that Fred's fanatic obsession with my sexuality was probably a result of his own repressed homosexuality. Now I can ache for him, but at the time I hated him. He threatened that if he ever even so much as suspected that I was having an affair with a woman, he would call the chief of my residency program (I had recently begun my residency) and tell him that I was gay.

I wasn't having an affair with anyone, but Fred's threat hung over my head like the sword of Damocles. Being gay was bad enough, but a gay gynecologist . . . Good Lord! I was sure I would be booted out on my ear. I still don't know what would have happened if Fred had actually called the chief and told him I was a lesbian. The chief and I had a very special relationship. I was his protégée, and he was my idol. He was like a father to me, and I adored him. He was the first doctor I'd ever met who clearly cared about his patients as people. Somehow he had managed to come through the medical mill without being mangled, and my being able finally to relate to patients as people had a lot to do with the chief. But I don't know what he would have done if he had known then that I was gay. Or maybe I think I do know, and just don't want to admit it. He was so accepting of me as a woman doctor, such a champion of me, that I still can't admit that he might have booted me out of the residency program.

Even now that I am a publicly identified lesbian, the chief and I have never discussed it. He's no longer with the health plan and neither am I, but I did hear, after I'd come out of the closet, that the chief told someone that he was "disappointed" in me. I knew the chief to be a mild man; for him to say he was disappointed in someone spoke volumes of disapproval. To this day the thought of his possible disapproval is still crushing, and perhaps hearsay had it wrong and I would have found him more understanding than I've been able to give him credit for being.

At any rate, the threat of public exposure via Fred was enough to keep me straight. From the time I began my internship until after I completed my board exams, I was unremittingly celibate. It wasn't until I was board certified that I felt secure enough to deal with my homosexuality.

My therapist was, fortunately for me, not into "curing'' homosexuals by turning them into heterosexuals. She did not think homosexuality was a disease. At the time this was a revolutionary position. It wasn't until 1973 that the annual convention of American psychiatrists decided to take a vote on the issue, and after a count of hands, decided (once and for all, I hope) that homosexuals are not sickos.

I continued my private therapy and also entered gay-oriented group therapy. I will be forever grateful for the support, nurturing and caring I found within that group. It was with them that I first began to tie the sexual knots inside me, which finally allowed me to understand why I was so terrified of my own feelings, even feelings that were not specifically sexual. My own guilty sense of myself had made me shrink from any and all emotional contact.

I will also be eternally grateful to my therapist. I can remember her standing before the group the first time we met and talking to us about homosexuality. She stood before a chalkboard and drew a horizontal line. ''This,'' she said, ''is the Kinsey scale. At one end of the scale''—she pointed to one end of the line she had drawn—''are the people who are exclusively heterosexual. They have sexual experiences only with people of the opposite sex, and their sexual fantasies revolve exclusively around members of the opposite sex. On the other end of the scale are people who are exclusively homosexual. Their sexual experiences, thoughts and fantasies are only with or about people of the same sex. In the middle of the scale''—and she drew a line at the midpoint—''are people who are bisexual. Their sexual experiences, thoughts and fantasies are about equally divided between the same sex and the opposite sex.

''Very few people fall at either extreme or right in the middle. According to Kinsey Institute research studies, only six percent of the population is exclusively heterosexual and only four percent is exclusively homosexual. The vast majority fall somewhere in between.

"As you can see from this scale, the actual behavior of people in our culture is at considerable odds with the culturally articulated norm. Our culture professes allegiance to the idea that the only socially acceptable form of sexual behavior is the strictly heterosexual, a 'norm' to which only six percent of the population actually conforms."

She delivered this whole lecture in a factual, value-free way, as if she were saying that a few rare people in our culture like only apples and a few like only oranges, and some like oranges and apples equally, but most have a mixed taste, liking both, some generally preferring apples but glad to taste an orange now and then, and others having more of a liking for oranges, yet experimenting with an apple occasionally. The trouble arose because the cultural rules ignored the facts.

The very tone in which she spoke was the beginning of an emancipation for me. I happened to be a lesbian in a culture that pays lip service to heterosexuality while secretly pursuing its polymorphous taste. My sexual orientation was not a dirty, wrong, bad and nasty thing, simply a matter of personal taste, and all my angst arose from this hypocrisy about who should like what.

I suppose I thought that being in a therapy group with gay people would be a matter of identifying the things that had "made" us gay. My therapist took the position that *why* we were homosexuals was beside the point. Despite all the learned papers and discourses and endless studies and theorizing, no one has the slightest idea why one person prefers sexual partners of the same sex while another prefers partners of the opposite sex, any more than we know why one person likes oranges and another likes apples. The business we had to attend to as a group was dealing with the terrible ravages wreaked upon us as homosexuals in a relentlessly heterosexual world.

Coming out of the closet is essentially a three-step process. First you have to admit to yourself that you're gay. Then you admit it to your friends and family. Then, maybe, you can admit it to the world at large. But the process is far from being easy or pat. It is wrenchingly painful in soul and gut, and left to myself I might have lived and died celibate and alone, dry and untouched. Or maybe not. Maybe that need to come soul to soul with another human being, open and eager, wet with wanting, was too strong ever to be extinguished by fear and shame.

Getting into therapy and into a therapy group of gay people was a big step in dealing with the internal aspect of my homosexuality. Now it was time to deal with the social aspects as well and, since by this time I was board certified and felt professionally safe, I did manage to take the first halting steps. In those days the only way for lesbians to meet each other was the gay bar scene. But I couldn't go to a gay bar. What if someone saw me there? Why, then they'd know I was gay. My terror of that eclipsed my sense of logic. It honestly never occurred to me that anyone who would have seen me in a gay bar would have been there because she herself was gay. Going to a gay bar was out of the question for me.

At the time, there was a newspaper in Los Angeles, *The Free Press*, that had started out as an antiwar-movement newspaper. Over the years it degenerated into a sleazy sex rag, but now the paper was just beginning its decline. It had a large classified ad section in which people advertised their sexual needs: "White, professional male, seeks female for close, loving relationship who's into whips, chains and bondage." That kind of thing. Gay people advertised in the paper as well, although they weren't allowed actually to say they were gay. You could advertise for a sexual partner who would tie you up, whip you, pee on you, but *The Free Press* had its standards: Nothing as perverse and sick as homosexuality could be mentioned in an ad.

Loathing myself as I did so, I responded to an ad that read "Professional woman in her mid-thirties seeking to meet with other such women." The woman I met through that ad was as predictably crazy as anyone else who advertised in *The Free Press*, but she did introduce me to the lesbian community. I attended a few parties and met a number of women, but I couldn't bring myself to get involved. Then one afternoon I got a call from a woman who explained that she had heard about me through mutual friends and understood that I was interested in athletics (which was true). She herself was an Olympic swimmer, and maybe I'd like to get together with her and have a drink or lunch.

I would and we did and we became lovers, beginning a relationship that lasted many years.

That was step one, coming out to myself. It took me five years to get to step two, admitting to my parents that I was a lesbian, and even then it was a matter of *admitting* it, as though it was something I was guilty of. I was living with my lover, and my parents wanted to visit. They'd been wanting to visit me for some time, and I'd finally run out of plausible excuses to explain why it just wasn't possible. So they were coming. If it hadn't been for my therapist, I think I might actually have hidden my lover's toothbrush and clothes and sent her packing for two weeks.

"Look, Jane," she said, "you're a big girl now. You've got to deal with mommy and daddy some day. You can't go on avoiding it forever. Do you really want to do this to a woman who loves you deeply? It's too cruel to deny her because of your own emotional cowardice." These were strong words for my therapist, who never pushed anyone through the

painful process of coming out. But she was right. I
had to tell them.

The letter was about ten pages long: I was gay. It
wasn't anything they'd done. It was just the way I
was, and I was happy that way. I was sorry about the
pain this might cause them. I loved them and was
afraid of losing their love. I still wanted them to come
and visit. Please. I put it in the mailbox and, feeling
terrified and alone, cried myself to sleep that night. I
was a grown woman, but there was still a lot of child
in me, and the child was petrified at the thought that
mommy and daddy weren't going to love her anymore. As a child you're dependent on your parents to
take care of you. Your very physical survival depends
on them. If they don't love and care for you, you
could, quite literally, die. Obviously, I was now able
to take care of myself, and I wasn't going to die if
they withdrew their love, but the emotional habit of
equating parental love with physical survival dies
hard.

I called my parents the next day. My father answered the phone, and I told him that I had written
them a very important letter. It wasn't something I
wanted to talk about on the phone. I wasn't sick or
dying or in trouble or anything, but I wanted them to
read the letter before they made their vacation plans
final. If they wanted to call me after they'd read it,
that was fine. I'd wait to hear from them.

My sister, Sara, called a couple of days later. My father had waited by the mailbox each morning to inter-
cept the letter before my mother could read it; he
hadn't let my mother know it was coming.

"Dad called and read me your letter, Jane," Sara
said. "He said he didn't know whether to burn it or
tear it up and throw it in the garbage.

"Jane, I've known for years that you were gay.
I guess I'm feeling hurt that you didn't trust me
enough to tell me, but I guess I can understand why.

Did you think I would love you any less?" She was crying. I was crying. "For godsakes, if two human beings in this crazy fucked world manage to find each other and share a little love, what does it matter whether they're purple, green, blue, Catholic, Jew, male, female, black, white. Jesus, I'm just happy you've found someone to love who loves you back." I never loved my sister more than at that moment.

Sara killed herself a few years later. She finished her nursing shift at the hospital one afternoon, picked up her paycheck, walked up to the seventh floor of the garage where her car was parked and stepped over the edge. I miss her still and always will, and perhaps the greatest regret of my life is that I was not there to catch her.

My parents did not come to visit me. I received an angry, hurt letter from my father. How could I have done this to them? Did I never think of anyone but myself? (How could I have told him that I was only now learning to do that?) He did not show the letter to my mother: "It would kill your mother." Guilt, guilt. There was so much guilt in my family, so much dark and killing guilt. It killed my brother. It killed my sister. It came close, at times, to killing me.

But it did not kill me, and I still am not entirely sure why. I think it was those three babies dying, and crying with the Harts. I think it was holding Alexa Kombronovich and, with her, crying again after too long denying my emotions. I think it was owning my own sexuality. I think it was quite simply refusing to die. I think it was, finally, digging beneath all that guilt and grime and finding a self that was mine; and once I found her I began to love her, love her fiercely.

ELEVEN

M Y MEMORIES of that part of my life are curiously indistinct, conjured up in images so wavering it is as though I am looking at them from underwater. I cannot remember exactly how or when things happened, but it must have been sometime during the aftermath of my coming out that I received a phone call one afternoon that, as theatrical as it sounds, really did change my life, although at the time it hardly seemed a momentous matter. The call was from a woman named Claudia, a member of a feminist group that was trying to establish a clinic where women could get low-cost abortions. She explained that the fees at the clinic would be on a sliding scale based on the woman's income level. In order to make this possible, the group needed doctors willing to volunteer their services.

Doing abortions was not my favorite pastime, but I still had a few noble ideas about a physician's responsibility to the community. I asked Claudia a number of questions about her group's setup, policies and procedures. I didn't want to get mixed up in something that wasn't medically sound. But she had all the right answers, and I offered to come down to the clinic the following evening to look things over. Claudia was delighted, and said she would schedule me for a training and orientation session at seven o'clock. I chuckled as I hung up the phone. I'd been through a dozen years of medical training, I was a board-certified physician, and they were going to train me in abortion procedures?—training session, indeed!

I was pretty full of myself as I left the hospital the next evening and headed towards the abortion clinic. There was the usual snarl of rush hour traffic, but I hardly noticed. I was too busy with my fantasies of the Great White Doctor ministering to the natives, too busy congratulating myself on what a swell person I was, a regular angel of mercy. I patted myself on the back and pulled onto the freeway.

The address the woman had given me was halfway across town. It wasn't exactly an upper-crust neighborhood, but that didn't bother me. Angels of mercy don't mind slumming; in fact, we kind of like it.

I found the freeway exit and headed south, as directed. I spotted the clinic's sign, parked around back and found the staircase that led to the clinic's rear entrance. I climbed the stairs and knocked on the door. No answer. I knocked again and waited. Still no answer. I knocked again and waited some more. I was beginning to get annoyed. I was *the doctor*. Doctors are supposed to keep other people waiting, not vice versa. Besides, this did not fit into my Great White Doctor fantasy. The natives were supposed to welcome me with open arms, not leave me standing in a cold, dingy back alley. I was about to stop waiting when the door was opened by a fuzzy-haired, harried-looking woman who said, "Oh, you must be Jane Patterson," with a marked lack of enthusiasm.

"I'm *Doctor* Patterson," I acknowledged, using the imperious tone of voice I'd picked up from a particularly pompous chief resident I'd known. I also put a bit of miffed in my voice so she'd be sure to know that I didn't like to be kept waiting.

It went right over her head.

"Well, come on in," she said impatiently, as though *I* was wasting *her* valuable time.

My Great White Doctor fantasy was rapidly getting ragged around the edges. The bit players had their lines all wrong.

I followed her down a narrow hallway to a small office where two women were madly typing away.

"This is Jane Patterson, the doctor," the woman said over her shoulder to no one in particular as, without pausing, she disappeared out a door on the far side of the room.

One of the women who was typing turned around and introduced herself.

"Hi, I'm Claudia, I spoke to you over the phone the other day. We really appreciate your taking the time to come down here like this."

This was more like it. I modestly mumbled something about being glad to help out. Claudia offered to show me around the clinic and led me downstairs to the waiting room. It was furnished with a couple of moth-eaten couches, a few grey metal folding chairs and thousands of posters and mimeographed flyers announcing consciousness-raising groups, child care programs and various and sundry protest gatherings—about what I'd expected. The operating and examining rooms, however, were a pleasant surprise. They were faultlessly clean and fully equipped. Claudia explained that what they hadn't been able to beg, borrow or steal had been purchased with a small grant they'd managed to snag.

"If you'll wait here a second, I'll find Gloria. She's in charge of new-doctor orientation and training," Claudia explained.

In a few moments Gloria and another woman, Patty, appeared and introduced themselves. Gloria explained that she was going to familiarize me with the procedure.

"I really don't think that will be necessary," I began, but Gloria ignored my interruption.

"We do things a bit differently around here."

A bit differently was right. While I'd been talking to Gloria, Patty had shucked her jeans and underwear, jumped up on the examining room table and hooked her feet in the stirrups. When I turned around, there she was, lying spread-eagled on the table, grinning up at me.

"First of all," Gloria continued, "we don't use drapes. Drapes are a tool of sexist oppression."

This seemed an exaggerated description of what was, after all, only a simple piece of white sheeting that doctors drape over a woman's knees during a gynecological exam. But it didn't sound as if Gloria was open to discussion on the matter, so I let it pass.

"They serve no useful purpose—which is not to say that they don't have a purpose. They do. They depersonalize the patient and mystify the simple process of gynecological exam. The gynecological exam can be compared to the rituals performed by priests and holy men in more primitive societies. All traces of personal or tribal identity are removed. The priestly attendant/nurse then drapes the supplicant/patient in the ritual robes and leads her to the altar/examining table. The woman is then placed in a vulnerable position— on her knees or, in the case of the gynecological exam, in the stirrups. The priest/gynecologist then makes his appearance and performs the magic rites.

"Just as the priest or holy man used ritual and magic to establish his authority, so the modern gynecologist"—Gloria gave me a pointed look—"establishes power over the woman patient by ritualizing the examination process. The traditional, authoritarian and paternalistic relationship between doctors and patients must be challenged. Women must confront the sexist medical profession head-on. We must throw off the bonds of oppression and regain control over our own bodies!"

Gloria delivered this lecture with the rousing air of one addressing a large crowd. As an audience of one,

I wasn't sure whether I was expected to say something in reply or simply applaud. The whole speech sounded rehearsed. (It was not until years later that I finally found out that Gloria had lifted her "rap" from an article by Belita Cowan on what she called the M.D.eity syndrome.) I was really at a loss for how to respond to all this, but Gloria solved my dilemma by plowing right on.

"So we advise women to fling the drape on the floor, and if the doctor tries to replace it, we advise throwing it down again."

I didn't like the way Gloria was throwing all this rhetoric in my face, but I was struck by the aptness of the doctor/priest imagery. Still, I had sudden visions of myself in an examining room, picking up a flung drape and politely and naively saying, "Excuse me, did you drop this?," only to be greeted by a white thunderstorm of reflung drapes. What would I do if my patients suddenly began behaving in this peculiar manner? I wasn't quite sure why the drape had to be flung. Couldn't the woman simply ask the doctor to disperse with the drape, or fold it up neatly herself?

At any rate, Gloria was dead right about one thing; drapes do tend to depersonalize medical procedures. Certainly, not having one made things more personal. The prospect of doing a pelvic exam with Patty, sans drapes, grinning up at me was disconcerting. I wasn't at all sure that I wasn't in favor of a bit of good old-fashioned depersonalization, no matter how oppressive.

Gloria slapped a speculum into my hand.

"Now," she said. "You will always call the client by her name, and you will explain every step of the procedure to her before proceeding. Show her the speculum"—she nodded towards Patty—"and tell her what it is."

Gloria was a real take-charge type, and remarkably effective. I began to suspect she was either a kindergarten teacher or a marine drill sergeant. I dutifully held up the speculum.

"Patty," I said, "this is a speculum."

"Call her Ms. Rousseau, not Patty," Gloria said haughtily. "She calls you Dr. Patterson, not Jane."

"Ms. Rousseau, this is a speculum."

"And I'm going to insert it into your vagina so I can see your cervix," Gloria prompted.

"And I'm going to insert it into your vagina so I can see your cervix," I repeated. "It won't hurt a bit." I was embellishing the script. Gloria did not approve.

"Some women find it a bit uncomfortable," she corrected, "but if you relax your muscles, it will be more comfortable. I'll go slowly, and you tell me if it feels uncomfortable."

We went through an entire mock abortion procedure, with Gloria coaching me each step of the way. It felt like the time in third grade when I forgot my lines in the class play and my teacher had to cue me from the wings. It did not feel good.

I beat a hasty retreat from the clinic that night, incensed. Who did those women think they were, treating me like that! I was a doctor, a board-certified physician. Not only that, I was a *woman* doctor—one of *them*. Gloria acted as though I was the enemy. I was doing them a favor, and they were insufferably rude. I wasn't going to have anything to do with people like that; they could just find themselves another doctor. They weren't going to have Jane Patterson to kick around anymore!

I don't know what would have happened if it hadn't been for Joe Foster. Joe was one of the other staff physicians at the hospital, and as far as I was concerned, he wasn't worth the time it takes to forget a bad idea. I suppose he was a good enough doctor technically, but he was a thoroughly repulsive human being. He was always patting nurses on the butt or sidling up to women and letting loose with some lewd sexual innuendo. He exuded an air of oily lechery that he apparently thought irresistible. Just being around him made my skin crawl. His conversation was always about pussies and twats and crotch rot and vagitch. A couple of days after the episode at the clinic, he caught up with me in the cafeteria.

"Hey, Jane, I hear you went down to that women's libber clinic the other night. They called me too. You know, I'm leaving here pretty soon to go into private practice, so I figured maybe I might get some business out of it. But Jesus, God I wouldn't want anything to do with that bunch of harpies. What a collection of cunts. You can't believe the things they said to me. Heard they gave you the business too. I told 'em to get fucked. Bet you told 'em where to get off too."

The idea that Joe Foster and I could be on the same side of the fence on any issue was enough to make me reconsider.

"As a matter of fact, I was quite impressed with the clinic," I said icily.

And the truth of the matter was that I had been impressed. Once my huff wore off, I had to admit that, like it or not, there was a great deal of truth under all that rhetoric of Gloria's. The thing that truly impressed me, though, was the ease with which I'd been able to do the pelvic exam on Patty. Normally women tighten up and clamp down when the speculum is inserted. They also tend to tighten their abdominal muscles when one hand is placed on the abdomen and the fingers of the other hand are inserted into the vagina and the rectum so that the pelvic organs can be felt. All this tension makes the doctor's job more difficult. Patty was considerably more relaxed, and my job was therefore easier. Even allowing for the fact that Patty was a pro, quite accustomed to having pelvics, it was obvious that if I explained what I was going to do to my patients before doing it, they wouldn't tense up as much.

I suppose that this great revelation should have been absurdly obvious, but until then it had never occurred to me. We were not trained to tell patients what we were doing, and I was still very much a product of my medical training. Like most doctors, I had learned to do pelvics by practicing on unconscious women about to undergo gynecological surgery. Once we mastered inserting the speculum and using our fingers to feel for any abnormalities in the contour of the pelvic organs, we graduated to performing pelvics on conscious women. Of course, we didn't bother explaining what we were doing to the unconscious women, but even when we were doing pelvics on women who were wide awake, we still didn't bother to say anything. For one thing, the doctor who was training us didn't speak to the patient. For a student to be so presumptuous as to do things differently from the resident would have been very bad form. Then, too, there's the embarrassment factor; it's not easy to carry on a nonchalant conversation with someone while your fingers are probing her vagina or rectum. But, perhaps the real reason we were encouraged not to talk to our patients during the examination was the fear that the patient would interpret the process in a sexual manner. We'd all been told tales of women who made sexual advances to their gynecologists. Our silence was supposed to keep things impersonal and nonsexual.

But as I thought about all this, I realized that although there are undoubtedly some women, and some doctors as well, who are so sexually confused that a pelvic exam becomes a sexual experience, such people are few and far between. Saying things like "This is a speculum and I'm going to insert it into your vagina so I can view your cervix" or "I'm using my fingers to push your uterus into a position where I can feel its shape by pressing on your abdominal wall" would hardly be considered erotic by most peo-

ple. Moroever, anyone who is so confused sexually as
to interpret a pelvic exam as a sexual come-on is probably going to do so regardless of whether the doctor is
silent as a stone or chatters away like a magpie.

But now I was no longer a student having to concern myself with aping the behavior of my mentor.
After having performed hundreds of pelvics, any social embarrassment I might feel was long since under
control. I was personally convinced that neither my
patients nor I were going to be thrown into erotic
ecstasy by some simple explanatory conversation during a pelvic exam. Yet I too maintained this curious silence.

Aside from anything else, simple human courtesy
should have led me to explain what I was doing before inserting a cold metal instrument into this very
sensitive area of a woman's body. Especially since I'm
basically a courteous person, why, when this simple
courtesy would make things so much easier for my
patients and for me, did I remain silent?

I didn't have an answer to this question. In fact, I
hadn't until then framed the question, but I think I
had already begun to sense that the women at the
clinic had things to teach me that would radically alter
my perception of myself as a doctor and as a woman.

Another thing about my experience at the clinic that
seemed, on the surface, even more trivial: I had been
told to address Patty Rousseau as Ms. Rousseau. Gloria had been quite haughty about it, like a society ma-
tron correcting me for a breach of manners. I thought
it just more of her lording it over me, but somewhere I
sensed her demand wasn't as trivial and petty as it
seemed. I generally called patients by their first
names; everyone did. Patients always called me Dr.
Patterson, never Jane. I had only a half-formed,
vague notion that this little detail of the form of address summed up the power relationship between a
doctor and a patient.

At any rate, when Claudia called later in the week to ask if I would come down to the clinic that Saturday to do abortions, I said I would. I told her I couldn't be there in the morning because I had to work at the hospital, but would come in the afternoon. Coincidentally, it was my Saturday to do abortions at the hospital. All abortions at the hospital were scheduled for Saturday mornings, and the staff took turns doing them. My turn came up every eight weeks or so, and here it was again. I wasn't thrilled by the idea of spending an entire day doing abortions, but I consented anyhow.

The procedure for doing abortions at the hospital was well organized and very efficient. On Friday afternoon the doctor whose turn it was to do abortions that Saturday would see each of the women scheduled for abortions. We did a pelvic exam to check the size of the uterus and make sure there weren't any physical abnormalities that might cause problems. We also took a medical history to make sure the woman didn't have any medical conditions that could interfere with the anesthesia. Then, assuming everything was okay, we gave her a consent form that explained all the possible risks and complications of the abortion procedure. We asked her to read and sign it and give it to the nurse. We also gave her a set of instructions that told her not to eat or drink anything after six that night, and to show up at the hospital at seven the next morning. All this took five or ten minutes. Generally it was the first time I ever saw the woman, and the last time I saw her conscious.

When I got into OR the next morning, my first patient was already in the operating room on the table, legs up, draped and anesthetized. I did the abortion, and then I scrubbed up, put on another sterile gown and went into the adjacent operating room, where another anesthetized woman was waiting. While I was doing the abortion on the second woman, the nurses took the first woman into the recovery room and got another woman on the table so that she was ready and waiting for me in the first room by the time I was finished doing the abortion in the second room.

At the hospital we used a general anesthetic. The clinic didn't have facilities to handle the complications that can occur when a general anesthetic is used, so they used a local anesthetic or, if the woman preferred, no anesthetic at all. Otherwise the procedure for doing abortions at the clinic was technically the same as our hospital procedure. But apart from the technicalities, there was very little resemblance between the way abortions were done at the hospital and at the clinic.

When I got to the clinic that afternoon I was met by the same woman who'd answered the door on my first visit. As enthusiastic as before about seeing me, she led me into a room where eight or nine women sat in a circle, talking. She took a chair out of the circle, set it down by the door and told me—told me, mind you, not asked me—to sit down. I was trying to think of something appropriately snotty to say to her when she turned her back on me and took a seat in the circle.

I sat down, thoroughly confused. I had come down here to do abortions, so why were they wasting my time with what appeared to be some kind of meeting? One of the women in the circle was talking, describing in step-by-step detail the procedures used to do an abortion. From time to time one of the other women would ask a question, and finally I caught on. Apparently this was an orientation session, and the women sitting around in the circle were the ones I would be doing abortions on. During our session the door opened and another woman came in and sat down. She introduced herself and explained that she'd just had an abortion that morning and was ready to go home.

"One of the women who had her abortion before me came in after it was over and talked to all of us, and it made me feel a lot better, so I thought I'd do the same thing for all of you," she explained.

"How are you feeling?" asked the woman who seemed to be in charge.

"Glad to have it over with," she said with a nervous laugh, and the other women asked her questions about how it had felt and how much it had hurt. One of the women in the circle talked about how nervous and apprehensive she felt. She was practically in tears. The others offered support and encouragement, touched her hand or gave her a quick hug.

The woman in charge passed around consent forms and read the form aloud to the group.

"This can sound pretty scary, hearing about all the things that can go wrong. We want you to be informed of the risks, but try to remember that these complications are very rare. Abortion is a very safe procedure. It's actually less risky than childbirth."

It was like having a bucket of ice water thrown in my face. I sat there thoroughly stunned. This was radically different from what went on at the hospital. We didn't explain to women what was going to happen during the procedure. Hell, we didn't even talk to them. There was none of this support or caring or concern. I sat there thinking of all the women I'd left sitting by themselves in examination rooms to read those consent forms outlining all the dire and even fatal complications of abortions.

I was also stunned by the realization that in a few minutes I was going to be doing abortions on these women, and they weren't going to be anonymous, unconscious bodies, but flesh and blood, very real people. I began to understand why they had made me sit in on this meeting, and it no longer felt like a waste of my time.

Then, while I was scrubbing up and getting into my gown, Gloria showed up.

"Now remember, you're to explain what you are doing each step of the way. Other than that, you needn't talk to the patient at all. One of our staff will be with the woman and will act as her patient advocate. Some women will have brought a friend along as well. They'll take care of the patient. You just handle the technical end. The advocate may ask you to slow down or even stop the procedure if the woman requests, so take your cues from the advocate. She's in charge."

I could feel myself starting to get hot under the collar all over again. Where did this woman get off talking to me like this? I was *the doctor*, and I was in charge, not some technician. Doctors run the show, not mere laypeople. Gloria acted as though I was nothing more than a pair of hands. I was thoroughly offended, but the whole afternoon had so completely shaken my notions of the proper sort of patient-doctor relationship that I couldn't get it together to argue with Gloria. I just did what I was told to do.

I came back to the clinic week after week. No one ever seemed particularly thrilled to see me, but I sat in my chair on the outside of the circle and listened each week, and was changed utterly by what I heard. I began for the first time to see how abysmally arrogant the medical profession was and how women were victimized by it.

I had thought that the liberalized abortion law was a "good deal" for women. The women at the clinic didn't think so. They were staunch proponents of "abortion on demand." The notion of women *demanding* anything from the medical profession was somehow threatening to me, but I came to understand things from their point of view. I remember one woman's story, told with a brittle humor.

"My friend told me about this psychiatrist who

would help me out. I made an appointment and showed up at his office one morning. He kept me waiting in his tacky, second floor walk-up reception room for an hour. Finally, he motioned me into his office and offered me a seat opposite his desk. As soon as I sat down he bellowed 'Penis!' at the top of his lungs—just trying to find out if I had any hang-ups about sex, he told me.

"After asking me a few questions about myself, he pronounced me 'more sensible' than the last woman who'd come to him wanting an abortion, a nurse who'd gotten pregnant 'while changing her pants.'

" 'Changing her pants?' I said. 'You mean the woman was a nurse and thought that you could get pregnant changing your pants?' I couldn't figure out what he meant.

" 'No, no,' he tells me, 'she was changing boy-friends and didn't know who to nail.' Nail meaning 'force him to marry her.'

"He spent the remainder of my half-hour appointment telling me about his next appointment, which was with a woman who packed her kids off to school in the morning, then painted her body with mascara and rubbed herself up against the furniture until she had an orgasm.

"This cost me two hundred and fifty dollars, but I consider myself lucky. I've known women who paid more and were propositioned by the doctor to boot. And all this just to be granted the privilege of being certified as crazy enough to have an abortion. If I apply for a job or for medical insurance and they ask me if I've ever consulted a psychiatrist, what am I supposed to say?"

In some cockeyed sense, this woman was lucky. I, too, had heard tales of exorbitant fees, sexual harassment and other humiliations. But, I realized, even when these sorts of things didn't happen (and I'm happy to say such abuses were the exception rather

than the rule), having to be certified as mentally unbalanced in order to be granted the right to control
what does or doesn't go on inside your own body
should hardly be thought of as a great piece of luck.

TWELVE

COMING TO realize that California's "liberal" abortion law was not the great boon to womankind I had thought was the first step in the political education of Miss, or rather Ms., Jane Patterson. It was not an easy course of study for me. I was one of the least likely, and certainly one of the least willing, candidates for any kind of involvement in the politics of the women's health care movement, or in any other movement for that matter. All I wanted was to have my own life work out with some semblance of order.

But over the next few years, as I continued to volunteer at the clinic once or twice a week, I was inexorably drawn into the movement. Actually, I was dragged in—kicking and screaming the whole way. And the women at the clinic certainly didn't see me as a likely recruit for their movement. For the first few months they regarded me with wary suspicion. These women were political activists, feminist radicals. They were waging war against the medical profession. I was a member of that profession, and therefore one of the enemy. But unlike most others in the medical profession, I was there. I was accessible. I drew a lot of fire.

Great emphasis at the clinic was placed on gynecological self-exam. In self-exam groups, women were given disposable plastic speculums and taught to examine their own vaginas and cervixes. The lay health workers at the clinic were also teaching themselves how to do pelvic exams on each other. Using a speculum is not terribly difficult; an adroit five-year-old could handle the mechanics of it. Doing a pelvic exam and feeling the contours of the uterus and ovaries is also fairly simple. Once the clinic workers began wielding the speculum on themselves and one another—and discovered how simple it was—they were even more furious with the medical profession. They'd been lying on their backs all these years, submitting to all sorts of indignities and paying large sums of money to doctors who supposedly had this specialized, intricate, arcane knowledge, and it was all a sham. They were as indignant as Dorothy and the Tin Man, the Scarecrow and the Lion were to discover the carney con man behind the awe-inspiring facade of the Wizard. I could understand their indignation. A gynecological exam *is* a simple matter, and doctors have made it seem more mysterious than it is. I too had played the con artist, and I suppose I deserved their indignation.

Still, indignation is indignation, and it was no fun being the target. Moreover, my ego was on shaky ground. I'd spent all these years of my life reaching after something I thought would make my life work, only to come up with a handful of nothing. I was thirty years old, and my life was supposed to be coming together. Instead I was a mess. My brother was dead. My sister was dead. My parents had disowned me. I was a lesbian, a weirdo nut case, in therapy trying to put the pieces together. I did not feel like a terrifically successful human being. But at least I had one thing to be proud of: I was a doctor, a board certified physician. And now the women at the clinic, with their denigration of the medical profession, were taking away my one remaining shred of self-esteem.

We might have reached an impasse if it hadn't been for something that happened at the clinic one afternoon. I was doing a pelvic exam on a woman who had missed her period and whose pregnancy test had come back positive. She was scheduled for an abortion, but when I examined her, her uterus wasn't at all enlarged. Her fallopian tube was, though: She had an ectopic pregnancy. The woman had already been examined by one of the clinic lay staff members, who mistook the swollen tube for the uterus and hadn't realized there was anything wrong. The tube burst, and we had to rush the woman to the hospital. It turned out she was a member of the health plan at my hospital, so I could do the emergency surgery on her there—and did. She needed transfusions, and the surgery actually was a life-saving measure. After that, there was a change in attitude towards me among the clinic staffers. Perhaps I wasn't a total con artist rip-off after all.

Maybe it was their change in attitude towards me that allowed for my change in attitude towards them. It had to do with the issue of the birth control pill. The Pill controversy was reaching its height about the time I first began volunteering at the clinic. It seemed that every time you turned around there was another "Is the Pill Really Safe?" article in one of the women's magazines. My initial reaction to these articles in the popular press was typical of most people in the medical profession, who found them "hysterical," "overblown" and "irresponsible." Of course the Pill was perfectly safe; we'd been told so in medical school. It was ridiculous to think that the drug companies would market an unsafe product or that the government would approve a drug that hadn't been tested and proven safe for everyone.

When the Senate convened hearings on the Pill, the medical establishment was thoroughly incensed. How dare the government interfere with the medical profession! The doctor-patient relationship was sacrosanct. Politicians had no business intruding upon it. We argued all this with a fervor and a righteous indignation reminiscent of those bigots who opposed desegregation on the ground that states' rights, not racism, was the issue at hand.

The attitude towards the increasingly alarming articles in the popular press was, well, maybe some women were complaining of headaches, nausea, depression and so on, but everyone knows how *women* are: You tell them that headaches are a side effect of the Pill, and they'll all get headaches. Then the English studies, linking the Pill to heart attacks, strokes and other serious side effects, came out. Most American medical journals reported these results with editorial comments pointing out that these studies were not conclusive; that the risks, if they existed, were statistically small. At my hospital these English studies were discussed; but these were, after all, *English* studies, done on *English* women, using *English* pills. The implication was that American studies would be more accurate and more reliable, and would vindicate the Pill.

Every time a new Pill scare article appeared, the women at the clinic would wave it in my face, spouting wild rhetoric about conspiracies on the part of pharmaceutical companies and the sexist medical profession. At first I pooh-poohed the whole Pill controversy. When anxious women came to me wanting to be taken off the Pill, I would reassure them, but after a while it became harder to do so. I remember a young woman coming into ER one night. She died of a blood clot on her brain. She was young, only twenty-two, and had been perfectly healthy. She was on the Pill. I took a closer look at the British studies and began to wonder.

I was shocked when the Senate hearings revealed that the first birth control pills had been approved on the basis of a study in which only 132 women in the study had been using the Pill continuously for a year or more. The women at the clinic were beginning to sound less crazy. Still, I wasn't ready to jump on their bandwagon. For me it was a choice between, on the one hand, the medical establishment with the full weight of rational, scientific authority and, on the other, this band of crazy ladies with their radical politics and their emotional rhetoric.

I remember arguing with a woman at the clinic one day. I conceded that the Pill could have dangerous, even fatal complications, but these side effects were rare. It wasn't fair to scare women as all these alarmist articles in the popular press were doing.

"My god," she said, "listen to what you're saying. It's okay to give women pills that might kill them, but don't tell them that. Kill them, but for godsakes don't alarm them."

Click. Something fell into place for me. If someone had told that twenty-two-year-old girl there was a very slight chance that taking the Pill would cause a blood clot in her brain that might kill her, maybe she wouldn't have taken it. Maybe she'd still be alive. I think that this was the first time I realized that the women at the clinic weren't asking to have the Pill banned. All they were saying was that women should be informed of the risks. All they were agitating for was a simple piece of paper, a package insert to be included with each box of pills, that would outline the possible risks and the side effects of the Pill. This didn't seem too much to ask.

I didn't become a "No Freak," a doctor who refuses to prescribe the Pill, but I did begin to inform my patients that its use carried certain risks and that the latest research indicated there were safer methods of birth control. Fewer and fewer of my patients chose the Pill or IUD's, and I became proficient at fitting diaphragms.

The Pill controversy began to undermine my faith in the medical establishment. The discussion of the Pill's dangers should have taken place in medical journals. Instead it had been the popular press that brought these dangers to my attention. The medical establishment simply didn't want to admit that there could be something wrong with the Pill. I certainly didn't want to admit that a pill I'd been prescribing for years could have serious and even fatal consequences, but that was no justification for the medical profession's see-no-evil-hear-no-evil attitude. It became clear to me that the medical establishment was more concerned with controlling population and maintaining their own reputation for infallibility than with protecting the individual women's health, hence their unwillingness to admit that the highly effective Pill might be less than totally safe for all women.

It seemed it was one thing after another in the early and mid 70s. First it was the Pill, then came the IUD. The intrauterine device, a tiny piece of plastic inserted by a doctor into the uterus to prevent pregnancy, was touted as being safer than the Pill; but it too turned out to have sometimes fatal consequences.

One particular IUD, the Dalkon Shield, was responsible for a number of women's deaths. Its "tail," the string that is attached to the IUD and protrudes into the vagina, was made of a number of filaments twined together. The tail apparently acted as a wick, drawing bacteria up into the uterus, causing overwhelming infections that sometimes resulted in infertility and even death. The Dalkon Shield was eventually banned, but there were also problems with other IUD's. They perforated the uterus, caused infections and sometimes resulted in ectopic pregnancies. Once again my attention was drawn to the dangers of a would-be panacea, not by my professional medical journals, but by articles in the popular press. And once again a birth control method that I had been told was perfectly safe turned out not to be.

The Dalkon Shield scandal was a particularly sleazy one. The Shield was codesigned by a doctor from

the prestigious Johns Hopkins University. Most
university-associated doctors donate their inventions
to a medical school for testing. But this doctor had
formed his own corporation to test, manufacture and
market the device. He published his results in a journal, identifying himself only as a researcher from
Johns Hopkins. Nowhere did he mention that he had
a financial investment in the device. The Dalkon
Shield was leased to a pharmaceutical company, and
glossy ads began to appear in the medical journals
quoting the research done at Johns Hopkins. The ads
claimed a very high effectiveness rate, higher than
that of other IUD's.

Seeing these high effectiveness rates backed up by
the considerable prestige of Johns Hopkins, I, like
many trusting doctors, began prescribing Dalkon
Shields. What the ads and journal articles didn't tell
us was that the women in the study in which there
were such wonderful effectiveness rates were not just
fitted with IUD's; they were also told to use
spermicidal foam on days ten through seventeen of
their cycles. It was not until the women at the clinic
showed me an article, "A Case of Corporate Malprac-
tice," by investigative reporters Mark Dowie and
Tracy Johnston, in *Mother Jones* magazine, that I was
aware of all this. The article further stated that there
was evidence that the company had been alerted by
one of its own employees to the problem of the tail's
role in promoting infection, and had done nothing
about it.

Drug companies had marketed the Pill without adequate testing. They had ignored the problems with
the IUD. Then there was Flagyl. Flagyl is a drug used
to treat trich, a common vaginal infection. The drug's
manufacturer had submitted the required testing
showing it to be safe, and the drug was approved.
However, independent testing later indicated that
Flagyl caused cancer in lab animals. When the FDA

reviewed the drug company's data, it found that the company had been either extremely careless or outright fraudulent in its presentation.

The claim made by the women at the clinic that drug companies were interested in profits even at the expense of safety no longer sounded like a wild accusation. I began to wonder if I could trust any of the drugs I routinely prescribed.

I really began to wonder after word got out about DES. DES, or diethylstilbestrol, is a synthetic estrogen. Beginning in the early forties, DES was given to pregnant women who had a history of miscarriage, premature birth, signs of bleeding in early pregnancy, or conditions like diabetes or hypertension that might lead to miscarriage or premature birth. The theory behind its use was that since the body produces large amounts of estrogen to support a pregnancy, giving these women extra estrogen would provide that much more support. Soon after, in a typically American "more is better" vein of thought, it was decided that maybe you could get even healthier, better-than-normal babies by giving extra estrogen also to pregnant women with no history of miscarriages, or any other problems. So DES was also given to women who were having completely normal pregnancies.

The drug was given, willy-nilly, to millions of women. Some of them weren't even told the truth about what they were being given, and thought that it was just a vitamin to help them have healthier babies. The medical profession was not in complete accord on this issue. In the early fifties a few doctors began to question the studies that suggested DES was effective in preventing miscarriages and would produce healthier babies. Those studies had not been very scientific. Women in one such study were divided into two groups, one of which received DES and the other nothing. The doctors who had begun to question the DES research argued that the seemingly superior results from the DES group in this study might have been attributable to the fact that the DES women were getting better prenatal care, more attention from their doctors and so forth. They argued that in order to get truly scientific results, a double blind, randomized, study should be done. In a double blind study, both groups are given pills. Some get the real DES and others get fake pills. Neither doctors nor patients know who's getting what, so the results of the study aren't compromised by such factors as extra attention.

The effectiveness of DES became a highly emotional issue among doctors. Finally a double blind study was done, and the DES group actually had higher rates of miscarriage and other problems than the control group.

That should have put an end to DES usage, but it didn't. The medical establishment continued to waver on the issue. The pro-DES group was centered at Harvard and the anti-DES group in the Midwest. It became a war of allegiances. If you graduated from Harvard or another eastern medical school, you were indoctrinated in the virtues of DES. If you graduated from a midwestern school, you were anti-DES and didn't prescribe it. I was subject to both points of view, but luckily I was young and idealistic and intuitive enough to feel that it wasn't right to tamper with the natural process of pregnancy. I never prescribed DES.

The debate died down, and doctors went on prescribing or not prescribing DES according to their background, training and personal inclination. Then on April 22, 1971, the *New England Journal of Medicine* published an article by Arthur Herbst and his associates that rocked the medical profession. Herbst had discovered seven cases of a rare form of vaginal cancer in young women. Not only was the cancer rare, it had never before been seen in a woman under the age

of fifty. After years of careful research, Herbst had
discovered that the mothers of all these teenage cancer victims had taken DES during their pregnancies.

Since that time, over three hundred other cases of
cancer have been discovered in DES daughters. And
in addition to cancer there are abnormalities in the
cervix, infertility and higher rates of miscarriage in
DES daughters. It was learned later that DES sons
suffer too, with fertility problems and abnormalities
in their genital organs.

It was a shock to realize the time-bomb effect that
carelessly prescribed drugs could have, but what was
even more disturbing was the failure of government
agencies to act on the information. The FDA had
Herbst's data months before they took any action.
In fact the FDA banned the use of DES in feed for
chicken and cattle long before they banned its use in
women.

A few years later, it was Premarin—another estrogen product. One might expect that the problems
with birth control pills and DES would have made the
medical profession a little less haphazard about the
use of estrogen. Not so. Estrogen replacement therapy was big business.

Estrogen replacement therapy (ERT) means giving
estrogen to women no longer producing estrogen in
their own bodies; either they'd had their ovaries sur-
gically removed or they'd reached menopause. We'd
been taught in medical school to think of menopause
as a disease, an estrogen deficiency disease. The drug
companies spent a fortune promoting the idea that
women needn't go through the rigors of menopause,
that they could be "forever young" if we'd just
prescribe daily estrogen tablets to replace the estrogen their bodies were no longer producing. The
most popular and widely used of these estrogen
products was Premarin. Though Premarin is effective
in treating hot flashes, it will not keep a woman from

aging. But no one paid much attention to this fact. Instead, doctors, spurred on by the miraculous claims of the drug companies, began prescribing Premarin and other estrogen products to all their menopausal patients, whether or not they were having hot flashes.

In all my years of medical training, I don't remember anyone ever questioning this practice—except Harry. Harry was one of the staff doctors at the hospital. He was there when I began my residency, and I worked with him once I joined the staff. Harry had a "thing" about Premarin. He thought it caused cancer of the uterus. He was generally regarded as a lovable eccentric.

During the weekly pathology conferences I attended as a resident, we'd look at slides or actual specimens of the tissue that had been removed during surgery that week. Every time there was a cancerous uterus, Harry would want to know, "Was she on Premarin?"

"Oh, Harry," everyone would groan.

One day Harry slipped and fell, and did something to his back. He was laid up for a week. While he was on his back, he conceived the idea of going back through the hospital records and pulling the files of all the women who'd been treated for uterine cancer to see if they'd been on Premarin. Harry was at it for months and months, and everyone treated his project with an amused tolerance, the way you might treat an odd-duck uncle who was building a boat in the basement.

Harry's ship came in. He wrote up his results and submitted the article to the *New England Journal of Medicine*. Harry's was the first article that linked ERT and uterine cancer, and it was swiftly followed by a series of studies that confirmed his findings. An alarming number of women who take ERT develop uterine cancer.

I could go on listing the shocks that reverberated through the medical world in the seventies but it's probably sufficient to say that they shook my faith in drug companies, in medical journals, in the entire medical profession, to its core. The women at the clinic no longer seemed like crazy ladies to me. They were right. There was something terribly wrong with the way the medical profession dealt with women. I jumped on the bandwagon and began to speak at symposiums, conferences and other gatherings.

Out of my disenchantment with the medical profession came a whole new way of dealing with patients. I could no longer play the Doctor-as-God role. The best I could do for patients was to tell them what I knew, to inform them to the best of my ability and let them make their own choices. It was, for me, a very different way of doing business.

THIRTEEN

I WAS often angry in those years, but it was a good
clean anger, a righteous anger. The early and mid
seventies were, by and large, happy years for me.
My personal life was working out, and I loved, truly
loved, my work.

My life was not, however, hout its contradictions. I was openly living as a lesb an. But although I
didn't try to hide my homosexuality, I wasn't pro-
claiming it from the rooftops either. If you'd asked
me, I wouldn't have lied about it. Still, I had not taken
step three in the coming out process—announcing to
the world at large that I was a lesbian. Not many people were willing to do that in those days, and with
good reason.

You could lose your job. The gay press was always
full of stories about gay teachers, gay military people,
gay government workers, who had been fired because they were gay. If people were uptight because
their kids' teachers were gay, I didn't imagine they'd
react very kindly to a gay gynecologist. My life was
going too smoothly to upset the applecart. But at the
back of my mind was the nagging voice of my conscience saying that I had a certain responsibility.

The world does not move forward without a little
push from courageous individuals once in a while. I
think here of Rosa Parks, one of my favorite heroines,
a black cleaning lady in Montgomery, Alabama, who
sat down in the only empty seat on the bus one eve-

ning and refused to get up and move to the Negro section at the back, thereby sparking the civil rights movement. I truly believe that the world could not continue to exist without these people, but I didn't want to be one of them, not even in some small way. Dammit, my life was finally beginning to work out! Why should I have to be the one? I whined at my conscience.

We all know how some people are born to greatness, others achieve it and still others have it thrust upon them, right? Well, there are yet others who simply bumble into—if not greatness, at least self-respect.

What I'm trying to say is that a woman I knew who was a writer for a gay newspaper asked me if she could interview me for an article in her paper, News West. I was too embarrassed to say no, but I wanted with all my heart to say no, and secretly cursed her for asking me. However, I felt I had a responsibility to other gay women. I knew how much it would have meant to me, just a few years earlier, to know there were other gay doctors, that there were gay people who were living full and happy professional lives. I also had a responsibility to myself: I was gay and I wasn't ashamed of it (well, hardly, anymore), so why did I have to live a constant lie? I owed it to myself to be true to myself. So I said yes.

Actually, my granting the interview was not as courageous as I might be making it sound. News West was an obscure paper. The only people who read it were gay, so doing an interview with them wasn't really very risky. Or so I thought. As it turned out, News West was distributed via those metal vending machine racks you see on street corners. There's usually a whole row of them, consisting of maybe one or two regular papers and a bunch of more obscure ones like The Free Press, a neighborhood newspaper, swinging singles rags and things like News West.

The issue came out with a picture of me on the front

page, emblazoned with a headline: "Gay Gynecologist Speaks Out." It was then that I discovered *News West* was sold in the row of vending machines right outside the main door of the hospital.

The official reaction was complete silence, but people did know about it. In fact, even though I knew that one out of every ten people in this country is gay, I was shocked at the number of people at the hospital who came up to me and said, "Oh, I saw the article in *News West*. I didn't know you were gay. How come I never see you at the Gay Community Service Center?"—or at this place or that place. Even people who were straight came up and said things like, "Gee, that must have taken a lot of courage." I tried to explain that actually I'd never suspected that anyone would see the article. But it was too late: I was the courageous gay gynecologist.

I suppose you are in the end what you pretend to be, and over the next few years I found myself becoming a gay spokesperson. There followed a round of numerous radio and TV talk show appearances. I was tapped to give the annual "Lesbian Sexuality and the Health Care Needs of the Lesbian Patient" lecture at the local medical school. I even made a TV special, which my friends refer to as the "See the Gay Lady Play Tennis Show." It was a program about gay people in nontraditional occupations, in other words on homosexual men who were construction workers rather than interior decorators, and lesbians who weren't marine drill sergeants. It was a kind of "day in the life of " thing, and a camera crew followed me around on a "typical" day. The idea was to present gay people as normal, regular people, instead of horned devils; people who did the same thing as "regular," heterosexual people. As evidence of my normality, they wanted to show me participating in some everyday activity.

"Well, what do you do in your spare time?" the director wanted to know. In my spare time I sit in a chair and stare blankly at the wall because I'm so worn out from working, but I didn't want to say so. He spied a tennis racquet in the back seat of my car. It had been sitting there unused for a good year, maybe two. Nothing would do but that they film me playing tennis. What could be more normal and regular! It must have taken them six hours to finally get what they thought might be acceptable film in the can, and I was stiff and sore for a week.

"That must have taken a lot of courage," people said after the special aired. I was too tired to try to explain.

About this time, I actually did do something that required, for me, a deliberate sort of courage. It had to do with another of the contradictions in my life. I was living a dual life. I was one kind of doctor at the clinic and another, very different kind of doctor when I worked for the medical plan.

If a woman came to see me at the medical plan, she met Dr. Patterson, who wore the requisite doctorly white coat. I would examine her without speaking to her, and afterwards, when she was seated across the desk from me in my office, I would tell her, calling her by her first name, what was wrong with her and what should be done about it. If a woman came to see me at the woman's clinic where I was now handling regular gynecological appointments as well as abortions, she was met by Jane Patterson, dressed in regular street clothes. I examined her, explaining in detail what I was doing. Then we would sit down together, on a couch or in armchairs around a coffee table, and I would explain what, if anything, was wrong with her. Then I would outline all the possible options for treating her, the pros and cons of each method of treatment, and would ask her what *she* wanted to do.

As time wore on I began to feel a lot more comfortable being Jane Patterson than being Dr. Patterson. I liked Jane Patterson better. There began to be a certain amount of absentminded spillover, and at the medical plan I would be Jane Patterson instead of Dr. Patterson. And sometimes I would deliberately leave my white coat behind and see my patients in my regular clothes. The nurse would come racing down the hall after me: "Dr. Patterson, Dr. Patterson, you forgot your coat."

I'd hate to tell you how long it took me to tell her that I hadn't forgotten my coat, I just didn't want to wear it anymore.

I might have been content to go on living this dual life except that within the medical plan, things were changing. The number of subscribers to the plan had grown astronomically. But the staff had not grown accordingly, so we were having to see more and more patients, which meant less and less time with each patient. No one else was complaining, though, so I didn't.

I was seeing patients in the medical plan's gynecology clinic one morning. Half the morning was already gone and the waiting room was still packed. I was behind schedule. I was always behind schedule in gynecology clinic. It was just routine stuff—Pap smears, pelvic exams, simple vaginal infections, contraception—but the patient load was too heavy. Too many appointments had been scheduled. I vowed to bring this up at the next department meeting, knowing at the same time that I never would.

It's me, I told myself. I'm slower than the other doctors. I'll just have to learn to work faster.

A young woman now awaited me in the examining room. I'd seen her in clinic before. She was a Mormon, and like many Mormons, she had a large family, six kids. She was in for her annual Pap smear and pelvic exam, which took only a few minutes. I considered trying to save some time by skipping the breast exam; it wasn't mandatory.

As I was examining her breasts, she said earnestly, in her broad country drawl, "Doctor, I know you're going to think I'm just a terrible person for saying this, but I got six kids and I'm only twenty-seven years old. By the time the youngest one is all grown, I'll still only be thirty-eight, and that's not old. I used to draw some and paint too. I haven't kept up with it, not with six kids and all, but someday, when the kids are grown, I'd like to get back to it."

She hesitated, then plunged on.

"I just don't want to live and die and all I can say I did was raise six kids. I want my tubes tied."

"I don't think that's terrible at all," I told her, and she relaxed visibly. Could she really have thought that I'd think her a terrible woman because she didn't want more than six kids? In this day and age, could she really have thought this? Yes, I answered myself, yes, this thought truly worried her.

I reassured her further and told her that, in my book, saying you've raised six kids in a single lifetime was saying a lot. I outlined the operation for her and mentioned the option of a vasectomy for her husband, vasectomy being a simpler and safer procedure than tubal ligation. She was amused by my ignorance.

"Merle? A vasectomy? Merle doesn't want no more kids, but he sure don't want anyone cuttin' on him, not down there." Clearly, she thought me a royal fool for even suggesting it.

I explained the procedure some more, answered her questions and had my nurse schedule an appointment at the sterilization clinic for her.

Now I was really behind schedule. I should have seen two or three patients in the time it had taken me to see this last one. I glanced out towards the waiting room. Still full. Out of the corner of my eye, I saw a little old man sitting by himself in the back of the room. He was gnomelike, wizened and shrunken, but there was something bright and lively about his eyes; they made him look like a leprechaun. At any rate, he cut an improbable figure in the gynecology clinic, which was otherwise filled with robust young women. Somebody's grandfather, I assumed.

My next patient was an eighteen-year-old girl about to leave home for her first year at college. She was also in for her regular gynecological checkup.

"Can a doctor tell whether or not a person's a virgin?" she asked, slightly anxious. I was to understand that she wasn't, of course, asking for herself; she had a friend who wanted to know. What she really wanted to know was whether I'd prescribe birth control for her without telling her mother. Delicately, I led the conversation around. She wanted the Pill. I told her that that was fine with me, but why didn't she spend a few minutes reading over these booklets describing the Pill and the other available methods of birth control? Then I brought the nurse in to talk to her.

If someone wants the Pill, I'm perfectly willing to prescribe it, but I wanted to be sure this young girl understood the risks as we know them, and was aware there were other options available to her.

I saw a few more patients, and by the time I got back to her, she had changed her mind.

"Do you really think I could learn to use a diaphragm?"

"Yes," I told her, "I'm certain of it," and I spent the next twenty minutes fitting her and teaching her how to use it.

Out in the corridor, behind the nurses's station, Dr. Goldsmith, one of the senior staff physicians, was putting on his suit jacket. He'd finished seeing all his patients and was ready to go to lunch. Dr. Goldsmith did not like me, and the feeling was mutual. It was nothing personal on his part. Dr. Goldsmith disliked me on principle: All women doctors were unreliable, inefficient and incompetent. On my part, it was entirely personal. I disliked him, first of all, because he disliked me. Then, too, there was the fact that he was always dropping snide comments about doctors who couldn't handle the patient load, while he himself was never behind schedule, and always looked so smooth and perfectly tailored and unruffled that he made me feel rumpled and harried and hectic in contrast, which I suspected he did on purpose.

"Running a little behind schedule, Doctor?" He was all oily concern.

I'd sooner have danced on my grandmother's grave than admit as much to Dr. Goldsmith.

"Not really," I lied, turning away to look out over the waiting room. The old man was still there, along with half a dozen women; probably all of them my patients. Once again I wouldn't have time for lunch.

In and out they trooped, the next several patients. I was a marvel of efficiency—quick, curt and to the point. Wham-bam, thank-you-ma'am gynecology. Dr. Goldsmith, eat your heart out. And then, finally, I was finished. The waiting room was empty except for the old man. I walked over to him.

"Can I help you with something?"

He got up slowly, with effort. He was very, very old. He extended his hand to shake.

"You probably don't remember me, Dr. Patterson, but I'm—"

As he was speaking, I reached out and took his hand in mine.

"Mr. Swartz," I finished for him. "Why, of course I remember you."

His face lit up with pleasure. He was delighted that I had remembered him. After all, it had been more than ten years. In truth I would not have recognized him. He was an old man all those years ago when I had first met him, and time travels harder and faster on the faces of the elderly. No, I would not have known him had I not touched his hand. Once I touched him, I knew instantly.

Memory is a strange thing. Most of the time when we remember, we are just efficient computers searching back through the storage banks of memories in our minds, stringing together bits of data to conjure up a rational recollection of how it was then. But if we summon up a memory through our senses, it is much more. Think of a memory triggered by a smell. How much more intense, all-encompassing an experience it is, almost a *déjà vu*. To this day, I have only to catch a whiff of *eau de violette*, my grandmother's cologne, and I do not simply remember; I am there again, clamoring about her feet as she braids her long grey hair in the dressing table mirror. The very feel and taste of the air about me is transformed in that instant's turning back. So, too, it is with memories triggered by a tactile sensation. Mr. Swartz had a degenerative collagen disease, scleroderma, that dries the skin and alters its texture. Touching the parchmentlike skin of his hand, I was transported instantly across the years.

The staff doctor, the resident and I (the intern) are making rounds on the acute medicine ward. We stop in front of Mr. Swartz's bed.

"We need to determine whether or not there's renal [kidney] involvement," announces the staff man.

Kidney involvement with scleroderma is serious business. If the kidney is involved, Mr. Swartz's prognosis will be very grave. There's nothing you can do for it, and Mr. Swartz will just go downhill, until, eventually, he'll die of kidney failure.

"Certainly," agrees the resident.

"Hmmm," I say, making a vague noise that could be taken for agreement. I have no idea whether we need to find out if the kidney is involved.

"We'll have to do a kidney biopsy," says the staff man.

"Certainly," agrees the resident.

"Hmmm," I offer.

"Have you had much experience with this procedure, Doctor?" The staff man is talking to me, me, the lowly intern.

I am standing at the head of the bed, behind the pillow, where Mr. Swartz can't see me. Wildly, I pantomime, "No. Never," shaking my head and holding up my thumb and forefinger to form a big zero.

"Some," I say.

"Fine, you can do the biopsy."

It is a perfectly barbaric procedure, involving a wickedly long, hollow needle that must be injected through the back into the kidney in order to snip off a piece of kidney tissue by means of a tiny cutting instrument inserted through the hollow needle. I push the needle into Mr. Swartz's back.

"Are you okay, Mr. Swartz?" I hate having to do this to this sweet old man.

"I'm fine, just fine," he says, wincing in pain.

I push the needle in farther, feeling it glide through the dermal and subdermal layers and fat tissue. I push harder to force it through the muscle.

"You'll feel a pop as it passes through the fascia, then a bit more and you're into the kidney," the staff man instructs.

I feel the pop as the needle passes through the fascia, the membrane that covers the kidney, and now I move oh, so cautiously. If I don't go far enough, I won't be able to get any kidney tissue. But if I go too far, I might hit a blood vessel or, missing the kidney altogether, hit the vena cava, the major artery of the area; or I might nick the intestines. I could, in short, kill Mr. Swartz.

My hands are stiff with care. My neck and shoulder muscles are drawn up tight, pinched by claws of ten-

sion; perspiration stains blossom beneath my armpits
and from under my breasts. I twist the biopsy instrument; its two tiny jaws, poised, I hope, at the outer
edge of the kidney, snap shut. I retract the instrument, withdraw the needle, and there it is, a tiny
speck of Mr. Swartz's kidney.

"All done," I announce triumphantly.

I am still congratulating myself as I sit enjoying my
dinner that evening, when my beeper goes off. Mr.
Swartz has begun voiding bright red blood. I stand at
his bedside as he writhes in pain. On a scale of one to
ten, kidney pain is a ten. The tiny ureters leading
from the kidney are screaming in agony as swollen
clots of blood force their torturous exit from the kidney. I have hit a blood vessel, and Mr. Swartz is
bleeding internally. In the operating room he is given
eight units of blood. I watch, praying he won't die, as
the surgeon removes the damaged kidney.

My prayers are answered.

The next afternoon at the Complications Conference, Mr. Swartz's case is discussed. I expect the
worst. I will be drummed out of the profession,
stricken forever from the roll of physicians. My career
is at its end. But, no, the staff doctor presents the case
in a matter-of-fact manner. A regrettable, but not in-
frequent complication of doing kidney biopsies, he
says. It's not my fault. I'm off the hook.

But it is not the only hook. Mrs. Swartz takes to
bringing me pots of chicken soup, replete with fat
matzo balls. I am looking a bit peaked and must eat
well, the wonderful young doctor who takes such
good care of her husband, who has saved his life, she
tells her children and grandchildren. They crowd
around, thanking me. It is the same with Mr. Swartz.
It is more than I can stand.

"Mr. Swartz," I finally say, "there's something I
don't think you understand. About the kidney bi-

opsy, the reason you had to have the surgery, the reason you lost your kidney—"

"Ach, shh, no." Mr. Swartz wags a finger in the middle of my nervous confession. "So much education and so silly. They put so many facts in your head, you can't think straight," he mocks me gently.

"You think I'm stupid? You think because I'm an old man, I'm dumb? I know better than you what happened. You, you're like my wife. She thinks she's in charge of life. One of the children has a cold and she moans—it's her fault, she didn't feed him good enough. 'No', I tell her, 'It's the germs. The air is full of germs. He breaths the air. He swallows the germs. He gets sick. It's got nothing to do with you.'

"But my wife, she thinks different. She thinks she's responsible for what happens inside the boy's body. Like you. You think you should be responsible for the way the blood vessels go through my kidney. You think you should be able to see through my skin and bones into my kidney.

"You think I don't know. I know. My wife she's a good woman, but very conceited to think she's in charge of everything, but a good woman. Like you, a good woman, and a good doctor. I know. Here in the hospital, I watch. I see how you are. I see what you do. I hear how you talk to the patients, how you treat us. You care, a good woman and a good doctor. But I'm an old man. Go away now with your foolishness, and let an old man sleep."

"Yes, of course I remember you. How's the scleroderma, Mr. Swartz?"

"Not so good, not so bad."

"How in the world did you find me?"

"My wife, she's here in your hospital." He leaned forward, dropping his voice. "Women's troubles," he said confidentially, a gentleman of the old school. "I hear them calling your name over the loudspeaker.

I think to myself, 'I wonder if that's her.' So I ask the nurse and, yes, Dr. Patterson is a lady doctor. So, I come over here to find out if, all those years ago, I was right.''

"Right about what?'' I asked him as we walked down the hall towards the elevators, enjoying each other's company. He was going down, and I was headed up to surgery.

"I am an old man. An old man likes to know he was right. So all morning, I sit there and I watch what happens, and I listen to the ladies. 'The doctor says not to worry,' they say. 'The doctor was so nice. She explained everything,' they say. 'Yes, she answered all my questions. Oh, she took her time with me, that doctor, such a good doctor,' they say. So, now I know, I *was* right.'' and he stepped into the elevator.

As the elevator doors were closing, he said, ''As a favor, for me, maybe you'll look in on my wife? Her doctor, a good doctor maybe, but you'll check on her?''

I did look in on Mrs. Swartz, but not as a favor, more as payment of a debt. I owed Mr. Swartz. He made me realize what I was allowing to happen to myself. I was touched to hear what my patients had to say about me in the waiting room, but too many times I was *not* allowing myself enough time with them. I owed it to myself and my patients to change that.

I went home and drew up Patterson's Manifesto. It contained a number of demands, but the main one was that the patient load be decreased. I planned to deliver my manifesto at the next department meeting. You must understand that in all my years at the medical plan, I had probably never said more than two words at a department meeting—and now I was coming in with a whole list of demands. Not only that, I decided to add an ultimatum. If something wasn't done about it, I was handing in my resignation.

I was scared to death. I was pretty sure nothing constructive would result, and I'd have to put my money where my mouth was and resign. Then what would I do? I was a publicly identified lesbian. Maybe the man in the street didn't know it, but I figured it was fairly well known in medical circles. Who would hire a gay gynecologist? I'd have to go into private practice. Nobody was going to ask a gay gynecologist to join their business. I'd have to go it on my own, but where would I find patients? There was already a glut of OB/GYN's on the market, and what with the declining birth rate, OB's in private practice were scrambling for business. How many women were going to want to have a lesbian gynecologist? I'd starve to death.

But even scarier than putting my career on the line was having to defend my point of view to a bunch of male gynecologists. They'd scoff among themselves. Sounds just like a woman, they'd say, talking about silly women things.

And it was true that the patient load wasn't so heavy we couldn't give proper medical care. It takes only a few minutes to do a pelvic exam or write a prescription for pills. What takes time is the other, human, side of the business. The problem was where to find time to inform a young girl of all birth control options, rather than just shoving the Pill at her; time to hold the hand of a cancer patient, and hug her and let her cry on my shoulder; time to explain all the pros and cons of the various treatment choices and help a patient make her own decision; time enough to allow a woman to overcome her fears and ask me about sterilization.

I presented my list of demands at the next department meeting, passing out Xeroxed copies. Everyone read in silence. As I might have predicted, Dr. Goldsmith was the first to respond. He described his efficient technique for seeing a contraceptive patient in three minutes, a surgery patient in five and a cancer patient in seven. He offered to work with me to cut down on my waste of time, and suggested that under his careful management the patient load for the entire department could be increased.

I thanked Dr. Goldsmith for his suggestions, but explained that it wasn't the time it took to perform the technical business of seeing a patient, it was having time to talk with the patient. I explained about the Mormon lady, and the young girl who wanted pills but ended up with a diaphragm. I went on and on talking about informed choice and what I thought constituted proper patient care. I spoke about the Doctor as God role, the ritualization of the examination—how we needed to drop that role and encourage patients to see us as regular human beings, how doing that would make for better health care for our patients. I felt as though I were speaking Greek. Patients making their own decisions? Patients as human beings? Providing emotional support to patients? I didn't feel like I was getting through. Further discussion of my proposals was tabled until the next department meeting.

The hospital grapevine was on full buzz. I felt that my proposals had fallen on deaf ears; but I was wrong. One after another, staff members came to me and thanked me for giving voice to this complaint or that. The nurses also thanked me. One nurse came up and said, "Hey, I hear you're thinking of leaving, you should talk to John and Greg. They're thinking of leaving, too."

John and Greg were two of the other OB/GYN's on staff. We had lunch and enthusiastically began to plan setting up a private practice together.

"Listen, I think there's something I should tell you before we go any further. I'm gay."

"Guess what?" they said, grinning at me.

I was ready for the next staff meeting, my resignation neatly typed up, but before I could get there to deliver it, the new chief of the department called me into his office. He had taken over the job a couple of years before, when my first chief left.

"Jane," he said, "I was very impressed by your analysis of the problems in the department, and I agreed with much of it. I haven't yet announced it publicly, but I'm leaving here. I've spoken with the administration and with the OB/GYN staff, and I'd like you to think about taking over when I leave."

I was stunned. I'd expected anything but this. Never, in my wildest fantasies, had I seen myself as chief. I would be the only woman department chief in the hospital. The medical profession had, in response to the women's movement, opened its doors to women, but you could still count on one hand the number of women who were heads of departments. Easily. I would not only be the first woman head of OB/GYN at the hospital, I would possibly be the first gay woman chief in the history of the universe. It was heady stuff. I would have to think about it.

And I did think about it, over and over. The power and the prestige were enormously seductive. I would be in charge, and able to make changes in the way things were, to strongly influence the way medicine was practiced. I almost said yes, but in the end I refused. For two reasons.

First, I realized that the situation wasn't truly solvable. The medical plan had started out some thirty years earlier with young, healthy subscribers, but those subscribers had grown older and had more medical problems. There were constantly more young, healthy subscribers coming in, but the demands of the older subscribers were putting a burden on the system. Costs needed to be cut, and I would be caught up in endless battles. At the same time I'd be trying to get more doctors to handle the increased patient needs, and I'd be an administrator responsible for cutting costs. It was a no-win game, and one I didn't want to play.

The second reason for my refusal was that I wanted to be a doctor taking care of patients. As chief, I would find most of my time being taken up with administrative duties. I wanted to care for people, not administrate them. I wanted to deliver babies and care for other human beings.

It had taken so many years for me to learn to care and feel and touch and be touched, and I loved it, truly loved it. Maybe someday I'd go into administration, but for now it wasn't what I wanted. It wasn't what I needed. So, on July first, 1977, I pulled up stakes and went into private practice. It is a decision I have never regretted.